Cotton and Williams'
Practical Gastrointestinal Endoscopy
The Fundamentals

Cotton and Williams' Practical Gastrointestinal Endoscopy
The Fundamentals

Eighth Edition

Catharine M. Walsh MD MEd PhD FRCPC

Associate Professor
Division of Gastroenterology, Hepatology and Nutrition
Department of Paediatrics, The Hospital for Sick Children
Temerty Faculty of Medicine, University of Toronto
Toronto, Canada

Ahmir Ahmad MBBS BSc MRCP PhD

Consultant Gastroenterologist
Wolfson Unit for Endoscopy
St Mark's Hospital (The National Bowel Hospital)
London, UK

Brian P. Saunders MD FRCP FRCS

Consultant Gastroenterologist
St Mark's Hospital (The National Bowel Hospital)
Professor of Endoscopy Practice
Imperial College
London, UK

Jonathan Cohen MD FASGE FACG

Clinical Professor of Medicine
Division of Gastroenterology
NYU Grossman School of Medicine
New York, USA

Peter B. Cotton MD FRCP FRCS

Professor of Medicine
Digestive Disease Center
Medical University of South Carolina
Charleston, South Carolina, USA

Christopher B. Williams BM FRCP FRCS

Retired Physician
Wolfson Unit for Endoscopy
St Mark's Hospital (The National Bowel Hospital)
London, UK

Videos supplied by Stephen Preston
Multimedia Consultant
St Mark's Hospital (The National Bowel Hospital)
London, UK

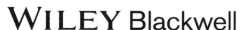

Registered Offices

John Wiley & Sons, Inc., 111 River Street, Hoboken, NJ 07030, USA

John Wiley & Sons Ltd, The Atrium, Southern Gate, Chichester, West Sussex, PO19 8SQ, UK

For details of our global editorial offices, customer services, and more information about Wiley products visit us at www.wiley.com.

Library of Congress Cataloging-in-Publication Data

Names: Walsh, Catharine M., author. | Haycock, Adam. Cotton and Williams' practical gastrointestinal endoscopy.

Title: Cotton and Williams' practical gastrointestinal endoscopy : the fundamentals / Catharine M. Walsh, Ahmir Ahmad, Brian P. Saunders, Jonathan Cohen, Peter B. Cotton, Christopher B. Williams ; videos supplied by Stephen Preston.

Other titles: Practical gastrointestinal endoscopy

Description: Eighth edition. | Hoboken, NJ : Wiley Blackwell, 2024. | Preceded by: Cotton and Williams' practical gastrointestinal endoscopy / Adam Haycock, Jonathan Cohen, Brian P. Saunders, Peter B. Cotton, Christopher B. Williams. Seventh edition. [2014]. | Includes bibliographical references and index.

Identifiers: LCCN 2023028999 (print) | LCCN 2023029000 (ebook) | ISBN 9781119525202 (hardback) | ISBN 9781119525189 (adobe pdf) | ISBN 9781119525158 (epub)

Subjects: MESH: Gastrointestinal Diseases–diagnosis | Gastrointestinal Diseases–surgery | Endoscopy–methods

Classification: LCC RC804.E6 (print) | LCC RC804.E6 (ebook) | NLM WI 141 | DDC 616.3/307545–dc23/eng/20231027

LC record available at https://lccn.loc.gov/2023028999

LC ebook record available at https://lccn.loc.gov/2023029000

Cover Design: Wiley

Cover Image: © David Gardner

Set in 8.5/11pt MeridienLTStd by Striave, Pondicherry, India

Printed in Singapore

M091782_301123

Contents

List of Video Clips

Preface to the Eighth Edition

In recent decades, there have been major advances in endoscopic techniques and technology. Improvements in endoscope resolution and image-enhancing modalities, as well as the emergence of artificial intelligence, are transforming endoscopic practice. The demand for endoscopy has never been greater. Yet, despite these changes, the fundamental principles of high-quality endoscopy remain constant.

Before exposing a patient to this invasive procedure, we must ensure that there is an appropriate indication and truly informed consent for it. Patient activity should be optimized to minimize any avoidable risk. The endoscopist should be skilled, or supervised if training, to ensure that accurate diagnosis and definitive therapy are performed with minimal patient discomfort or anxiety. When adverse events occur, they must be quickly recognized and appropriately managed.

It is a huge honor, and responsibility, to take forward the incredible legacy of Peter Cotton and Christopher Williams, the pioneering authors of this textbook first published in 1980. It is their commitment and dedication to the field of endoscopy that has made this text an invaluable resource for endoscopists all over the world. We are very grateful for their support, feedback and endorsement of this revised edition. The key word in the title, "Fundamentals," encapsulates the essence and differentiating aspect of this book. For decades, it has served to guide novices through their early days of learning to perform high-quality endoscopy. It remains focused on helping those in their first few years of experience advance more quickly along the endoscopic learning curve through competency toward excellence.

In this eighth edition of *Practical Gastrointestinal Endoscopy: The Fundamentals*, we have made updates and enhancements to reflect current practice to ensure that the text remains relevant and accessible for future generations of endoscopists. In doing so, we hope to maintain the original vision of Peter Cotton and Christopher Williams to help make skillful endoscopy easier and safer, ultimately improving patient care.

October 2023
Catharine M. Walsh
Ahmir Ahmad
Brian P. Saunders
Jonathan Cohen

Preface to the First Edition

This book is concerned with endoscopic techniques and says little about their clinical relevance. It does so unashamedly because no comparable manual was available at the time of its conception and because the explosive growth of endoscopy has far outstripped facilities for individual training in endoscopic technique. For the same reason we have made no mention of rigid endoscopes (oesophagoscopes, sigmoidoscopes and laparoscopes) which rightly remain popular tools in gastroenterology, nor have we discussed the great potential of the flexible endoscope in gastrointestinal research.

Our concentration on techniques should not be taken to denote a lack of interest in results and real indications. As gastroenterologists we believe that procedures can only be useful if they improve our clinical management; clever techniques are not indicated simply because they are possible, and some endoscopic procedures will become obsolete with improvements in less invasive methods. Indeed we are moving into a self-critical phase in which the main interest in gastrointestinal endoscopy is in the assessment of its real role and cost-effectiveness.

Gastrointestinal endoscopy should be only one of the tools of specialists trained in gastrointestinal disease—whether they are primarily physicians, surgeons or radiologists. Only with broad training and knowledge is it possible to place obscure endoscopic findings in their relevant clinical perspective, to make realistic judgements in the selection of complex investigations from different disciplines, and to balance the benefits and risks of new therapeutic applications. Some specialists will become more expert and committed than others, but we do not favor the widespread development of pure endoscopists or of endoscopy as a subspecialty.

Skillful endoscopy can often provide a definitive diagnosis and lead quickly to correct management, which may save patients from months or years of unnecessary illness or anxiety. We hope that this little book may help to make that process easier and safer.

April 1979
Peter B. Cotton
Christopher B. Williams

Acknowledgments

The authors are grateful to the dedicated collaborators who have embellished or enabled the production of this book. The artistic prowess and great patience of David Gardner has been crucial in enhancing the drawings and figures in this edition and several previous ones. The skills of Steve Preston have been invaluable in producing the online videos. The authors appreciate the input of Catherine Bauer from a nursing perspective in reviewing several chapters. At Wiley publishers, the guidance of Mandy Collison and Moyuri Handique's formidable editorial talents have made the production process seamless and even enjoyable. The authors also wish to register indebtedness to their respective life-partners (Geoff, Amina, Annie, Cori, Marion, and Christina) for their unending support—despite intrusions into personal and family time.

About the Companion Website

This book is accompanied by a website:

www.wiley.com/go/cottonwilliams8e

The website includes:

- 40 videos showing procedures described in the book
- All videos are referenced in the text where you see this logo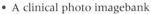
- A clinical photo imagebank

CHAPTER 1

Welcome to Endoscopy

If you are reading this book, you have likely just embarked on a journey to master the art and science of gastrointestinal endoscopy. Many of the experienced teachers you encounter along the way will sail through their examinations as if the scope is an extension of their hands, with a myriad of unconscious maneuvers and fast-thinking visual processing of what appears on the screen. They will make what appear to you to be near-instantaneous assessment and judgment calls as to how to respond to the information that comes into view. It can be easy for them to forget the wonderment of the first exposure to endoscopy that drew them into the field and now hopefully excites you to follow suit. At the same time, it is understandable for you to feel a bit overwhelmed by the apparent magnitude of the challenge you face to reach their level of proficiency.

Here are some reassuring thoughts to accompany your introduction to endoscopy. With time, practice, self-challenge, reflection, good role models, and feedback, you will be able to master what initially appears so daunting. By breaking down the many technical, cognitive, and non-technical skills into the components detailed in this book, and with equal doses of patience and persistence, becoming a high-quality endoscopist is well within your reach. Knowing that you will eventually develop the skills is comforting, but another source of support is the many resources available to you to make this learning trajectory far less bumpy and more expeditious. Several of these are listed at the end of this chapter. Hopefully, this book on the *fundamentals* of endoscopy will demystify the first steps of the learning process for you by clearly outlining the skills to learn and will make the path forward far less intimidating.

What general skills, knowledge, and mindset do you need to best set off to learn endoscopy? Contrary to common belief, you do not need to be a master video gamer or star athlete with already honed hand-eye coordination, although such skills may come in handy early in the learning curve for technical skills. Perhaps the most essential ingredient is having eagerness and motivation to learn. In doing so, you will also need to combine parallel threads of knowledge. This characteristic of endoscopy education is common to all medical specialties and highlights the importance of building one's fund of knowledge and making connections within it. You will no doubt have some of this understanding when you start to learn endoscopy, but the key to making progress is to use the circumstances

Cotton and Williams' Practical Gastrointestinal Endoscopy: The Fundamentals, Eighth Edition.
Catharine M. Walsh, Ahmir Ahmad, Brian P. Saunders, Jonathan Cohen, Peter B. Cotton, and Christopher B. Williams.
© 2024 John Wiley & Sons Ltd. Published 2024 by John Wiley & Sons Ltd.
Companion website: www.wiley.com/go/cottonwilliams8e

of each patient endoscopic encounter to augment your knowledge as it relates to the particular case at hand.

The technical skills required to navigate the endoscopic instruments and accessories, covered in detail in subsequent chapters in this book, are a second layer of knowledge that must be learned via observation, demonstration, deconstruction into component maneuvers, practice, feedback, reflection, and refinement. You will find this aspect to be novel and to require your full attention in the early phase of learning. A common mistake of teachers is to overload clinical training with lessons about visual image interpretation while a novice is focusing on mastering the basic manipulative physical aspects of performing endoscopy. Key to success in this effort is the attitude and understanding that progress is incremental, and one can *always* improve. Great teachers are themselves always striving to refine their skills and asking themselves the question "How can I do better?" Once you find yourself successfully completing components of the technical procedures without assistance, avoid complacency and push yourself to perform them better: more precise movements, less loop formation in the colon, smoother intubation of the oropharynx, etc. This will be the way to excel at endoscopy. Expertise is not innate; it is achieved by continually engaging in *deliberate* practice that is purposeful, feedback-informed, and conducted with the specific goal of improving performance.

The next major novel frontier for the student of endoscopy is re-learning how to look at images. By the time a prospective endoscopist passes an endoscope for the first time, the mechanics of assessing visual inputs has long since become automatic and immediate. For instance, imagine a hike through a forest. As you walk along the trail, you may notice some of the rocks and trees and the occasional bird as you pass by, but seldom do you stop and analyze the frames presented as you pass to truly notice patterns, assess the content, discern when something stands out as novel or atypical from the norm, decide what that unusual feature might signify, and choose whether to take a photo (or sample) or move on. Unless you happen to be a naturalist, you have probably become used to viewing your surroundings in a much more passive manner.

As you begin your endoscopy education, you will find it advantageous to consciously change the *way* you look. In the endoscopy suite, when your trainer asks you what you see on the screen, resist the temptation to blurt out a label or an interpretation, but rather start with a simple description. This requires you to notice and appreciate the features—the color, the contours, changes in the surface pattern, and the topography of the surface layer (bumpy or smooth, raised or depressed). Even when you learn the features associated with normal versus abnormal mucosa in various organs and with specific pathological diagnoses, pattern recognition begins with detailed observation and appreciation of the images that come into view. This is a learned skill that can be overlooked in the rush to label and correctly name what you see. Once you characterize the features, you will start to match what you are seeing to what you expect to find in a particular organ under normal circumstances and in various common disease states. This analytical type of data collection and processing is no different from that used by a novice botany student learning to recognize and name the vegetation along a hike through the forest. With practice, you will rapidly be able to detect when something is abnormal and figure out what the abnormality is. You will learn, too, how to respond to what you see as you progress in your cognitive skill development. Just as important a habit to form at the beginning of your training is a meticulous tendency to inspect completely and leave no blind spots in your examinations. To some extent, this overlaps with the technical skills required to maneuver your endoscope to visualize any hard-to-reach areas. The chapters in this book will guide you in how best to do this. However, the diligence that drives you not to overlook any area, and to go back and reinspect regions that you did not get a great look at the first time around, is a critically important practice.

As you get your first exposure to patients undergoing endoscopy, whether initially as an observer or with scope in hand, be mindful of everything happening in the suite. When you are observing a case in which the instructor is handling the endoscope, the tendency is to stare intently at the video monitor to see what the scope is imaging. However, it is often equally or more important to notice what your teacher is doing with their hands. Another key aspect to appreciate is how they are communicating and interacting with the rest of the staff in the suite. We all learn by reading, watching, listening to verbal instructions, and manually practicing and refining skills by tactile feedback. Trainees rely on each of these modes of learning to varying extents. You will soon figure out what works best for you.

Once you come to appreciate the magnitude of the different technical, cognitive, and non-technical skills you must master to perform high-quality endoscopy, you may again become overwhelmed. You certainly cannot learn all the skills at once, and the concept of cognitive overload will be discussed later in this book. A good rule of thumb that will help keep you on track and avoid becoming disheartened is to ensure that each procedure in which you participate provides you with at least one take-home lesson or opportunity to improve one skill, technical, non-technical, cognitive, or otherwise. After each case, review in your mind or with your trainer what you have just learned. Focused feedback discussions are essential to promote learning. Before each case, ensure that you set one to two learning goals, which may need to be adjusted depending on what you encounter during the actual procedure. For example, if you hoped to work on passing a gastroscope into the duodenum, but the patient has a large ulcer in the stomach, the main lessons from the case will necessarily deviate from the original plan. You may still try to achieve duodenal intubation, but the educational value of the experience will shift according to the circumstances that arise. This opportunity-based education is in contrast to a didactic A-to-Z learning agenda and remains an exciting aspect of proctored live endoscopy performance as a principal teaching tool in endoscopy.

You will soon appreciate that learning to perform endoscopy is a highly iterative process. Repetition, reflection, assessment, feedback, and monitoring progress are key features. You will notice that your best teachers will not only enjoy teaching but will themselves still be striving to continually improve and learn throughout their career. You will also see that they are always thinking about the patient and putting patient care first. Keeping these attitudes foremost in mind will serve you well, both as you learn to become an excellent endoscopist and as you progress throughout your professional career.

If this "welcome to endoscopy" seems to be more of a pep talk, well . . . that is what this is!

Resources and links

Websites
There is a huge amount of valuable material on the internet, posted largely by the main endoscopy societies around the world. These include many thoughtful guidelines for practice and training.

The main (Western) society resources are:
- American College of Gastroenterology (ACG): www.gi.org
- American Gastroenterological Association (AGA): www.gastro.org
- American Society for Gastrointestinal Endoscopy (ASGE): www.asge.org
- British Society of Gastroenterology (BSG): www.bsg.org.uk
- Canadian Association of Gastroenterology (CAG): www.cag-acg.org
- European Society for Gastrointestinal Endoscopy (ESGE): www.esge.com
- European Society for Paediatric Gastroenterology, Hepatology and Nutrition (ESPGHAN): www.espghan.org
- North American Society for Pediatric Gastroenterology, Hepatology and Nutrition (NASPGHAN): www.naspghan.org
- Society of American Gastrointestinal and Endoscopic Surgeons (SAGES): www.sages.org
- World Endoscopy Organization (WEO): www.worldendo.org

Online endoscopy educational resources include:
- American Society for Gastrointestinal Endoscopy (ASGE) core curricula: www.asge.org
- European Society for Gastrointestinal Endoscopy (ESGE) core curricula: www.esge.com
- ImageSIM (endoscopy image cognitive simulation tool): www.imagesim.com
- The Gastrointestinal Endoscopy Quality and Safety (GIEQs) Foundation: www.gieqs.com

Endoscopy books
Adler DG. *Upper Endoscopy for GI Fellows*. Cham, Switzerland: Springer International Publishing, 2017.

Chandrasekhara V, Elmunzer BJ, Khashab MA, Muthusamy VR. *Clinical Gastrointestinal Endoscopy* (3rd edition). Philadelphia, PA: Elsevier, 2019.

Chun HJ, Yang SK, Choi MG. *Clinical Gastrointestinal Endoscopy: A Comprehensive Atlas* (2nd edition). Singapore: Springer Singapore, 2018.

Cohen J. *Comprehensive Atlas of High-Resolution Endoscopy and Narrowband Imaging* (2nd edition). Chichester, United Kingdom: Wiley Blackwell, 2017.

Cohen J. *Successful Training in Gastrointestinal Endoscopy* (2nd edition). Hoboken, NJ: John Wiley & Sons, 2022.

Gershman G, Thomson M. *Practical Pediatric Gastrointestinal Endoscopy* (3rd edition). Hoboken, NJ: Wiley Blackwell, 2021.

Schiller KFR, Cockel R, Hunt RH, Warren BF. *Atlas of Gastrointestinal Endoscopy and Related Pathology* (2nd edition). Oxford, United Kingdom: Blackwell Science, 2002.

Schoenwolf GC, Bleyl SB, Brauer PR, Francis-West PH. *Larsen's Human Embryology* (6th edition). Philadelphia, PA: Elsevier, 2021.

Wallace MB, Fockens P, Sung JJY. *Gastroenterological Endoscopy* (3rd edition). New York, NY: Thieme, 2018.

Wang TC, Camilleri M. *Yamada's Atlas of Gastroenterology* (6th edition). Hoboken, NJ: John Wiley & Sons, 2022.

Waye JD, Aisenberg J, Rubin PH. *Practical Colonoscopy*. Chichester, United Kingdom: John Wiley & Sons, 2013.

Waye JD, Rex DK, Williams CB. *Colonoscopy: Principles and Practice* (2nd edition). Hoboken, NJ: Wiley Blackwell, 2009.

Wilcox CM, Muñoz-Navas M, Sung JJY. *Atlas of Clinical Gastrointestinal Endoscopy* (3rd edition). Philadelphia, PA: Saunders Elsevier, 2012.

Journals with major endoscopy focus

American Journal of Gastroenterology. Official journal of the American College of Gastroenterology.

Digestive Endoscopy. Official journal of the Japan Gastroenterological Endoscopy Society.

Endoscopy. Official journal of the European Society of Gastrointestinal Endoscopy, and 20 affiliated national societies.

Gastrointestinal Endoscopy. The official journal of the American Society for Gastrointestinal Endoscopy.

Gastrointestinal Endoscopy Clinics of North America. Quarterly publication of state-of-the-art reviews on the use of endoscopic procedures for the diagnosis and treatment of digestive diseases.

Gut. Official journal of the British Society of Gastroenterology.

Journal of Pediatric Gastroenterology and Nutrition. Official journal of the North American Society for Pediatric Gastroenterology, Hepatology and Nutrition and European Society for Paediatric Gastroenterology, Hepatology and Nutrition.

Surgical Endoscopy. Official journal of the Society of American Gastrointestinal Endoscopic Surgeons and European Association for Endoscopic Surgery.

CHAPTER 2

The Endoscopy Unit, Staff, and Management

Most endoscopists, and especially beginners, focus on the individual endoscopic procedures and have little appreciation of the extensive infrastructure that is necessary for efficient and safe activity. From humble beginnings in adapted single rooms, most of us are lucky enough now to work in large units with multiple procedure rooms full of complex electronic equipment, with additional space dedicated to preparation, recovery, and reporting.

Endoscopy is a team activity, requiring the collaborative talents of many people with different backgrounds and training. It is difficult to overstate the importance of appropriate facilities and adequate professional support staff, to maintain patient comfort and safety, and to optimize clinical outcomes.

Endoscopic procedures can be performed almost anywhere when necessary (e.g. in an intensive care unit), but the vast majority take place in purpose-designed "endoscopy units."

Endoscopy units

Details of endoscopy unit design are beyond the scope of this book, but certain principles are important to understand.

There are two types of endoscopy units:

• *Stand-alone, office-based procedure facilities* (called ambulatory endoscopy or surgical centers in North America) that deal mainly with healthy (or relatively healthy) outpatients, and generally resemble cheerful modern dental suites.

• *Hospital-based units* which must also provide a safe environment for managing sick inpatients, more complex procedures, such as endoscopic retrograde cholangiopancreatography (ERCP), and the whole range of therapeutic techniques. These units more closely resemble operating suites.

Functional planning

Units that serve both the above functions should be designed to separate patient flows as far as possible. The modern unit has areas designed for many different functions. Like a hotel or an airport (or a Victorian household), the endoscopy unit should

Cotton and Williams' Practical Gastrointestinal Endoscopy: The Fundamentals, Eighth Edition.
Catharine M. Walsh, Ahmir Ahmad, Brian P. Saunders, Jonathan Cohen, Peter B. Cotton, and Christopher B. Williams.
© 2024 John Wiley & Sons Ltd. Published 2024 by John Wiley & Sons Ltd.
Companion website: www.wiley.com/go/cottonwilliams8e

have a smart public face ("upstairs"), and a more functional back hall ("downstairs"). From the patient's perspective, the suite consists of areas devoted to reception, preparation, procedure, recovery, and discharge. Supporting these activities are many other "back hall" functions, which include scheduling, endoscope reprocessing, preparation, maintenance and storage of equipment, reporting and archiving, education and training, and staff management.

There should be spheres of activity for the endoscopist and assistants, as well as clean and dirty regions. One side of the room should be dedicated to endoscopy assistants who have easy access to accessories, supplies, and medications in cabinets directly behind them. On the other side of the room, the endoscopist should have a hand-washing area and workstation available to them. If anesthesia is used, the associated medication and supplies should be located at the head of the bed.

Procedure rooms

The rooms used for endoscopic procedures should:
- *not be cluttered or intimidating* as most patients are not sedated when they enter, so it is better for the room to feel warm and comfortable rather than like an operating room.
- *be large enough* to allow a patient stretcher/trolley to be rotated on its axis, and to accommodate all of the equipment and staff (and any emergency team), but also compact enough for efficient function.
- *be laid out with function in mind*, keeping nursing, endoscopist, and anesthesiologist (when present) spheres of activity separate (Fig 2.1), and minimizing exposed trailing electrical cables and pipes (best by ceiling-mounted beams).

Each room should have:
- *piped oxygen, CO_2, suction, a water supply, and electrical outlets for ancillary equipment*;

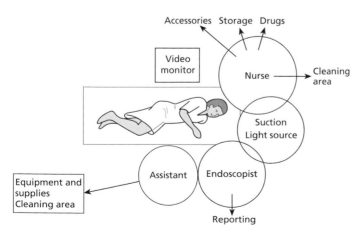

Fig 2.1 Functional planning—showing logical separation of the spheres of activity for endoscopy team members.

- *lighting* planned to illuminate nursing activities but not over-stimulate the patient or disrupt the endoscopist's line of vision;
- *adjustable video monitors* placed ergonomically, directly in front of the endoscopist to allow for neutral neck and back postures, with adjustable height and location to accommodate varying heights and the endoscopist's preferred viewing distance, ideally one on each side of the patient to allow all staff to view and respond during the procedure and enable the patient to view, if wished;
- *adequate counter space* for accessories, with hand-washing facilities and a large sink or receptacle for dirty equipment;
- *storage space* for equipment, supplies, and medications required on a daily basis to assure items are available when needed;
- *systems of communication* with the charge nurse desk, and emergency call;
- *workstation with computer system* that enables data capture and management, recording and reporting of endoscopic procedures and audit of quality indicators, and, ideally, is integrated into the electronic health record system;
- *two doors* to allow for easy access and simultaneous entry of clean instruments and removal of used equipment;
- *disposal systems* for hazardous materials.

Units serving children should have age/size/weight-appropriate equipment and pediatric-specific, patient- and family-centered processes for pre-procedure and recovery phases of care with a goal to reduce anxiety and provide age-appropriate care.

Patient preparation and recovery areas

Patients need a private place for initial preparation (undressing, safety checks, intravenous [IV] access), and a similar place in which to recover from any sedation or anesthesia. In some units these functions are separate, but can be combined to maximize flexibility. Many units have simple curtained bays, but rooms with solid side walls and a movable front curtain or door are preferable. They should be large enough to accommodate at least two people in addition to the patient on the stretcher, and all necessary monitoring equipment.

The "prep and/or recovery bays" should be adjacent to a central nursing workstation. Like the bridge of a ship, this is where the nurse captain of the day controls and steers the whole operation, and from which recovering patients can be monitored.

All units should have at least one private room for sensitive interviews/consultations before and after procedures.

Negative pressure rooms are preferred to help mitigate infection-related risks, particularly related to coronavirus disease 2019 (COVID-19), and to permit efficient air changeover between procedures. In resource-limited settings, industrial-grade high-efficiency particulate (HEPA) filters may be a reasonable alternative.

Equipment management and storage

There must be designated areas for endoscope and accessory reprocessing, and storage of medications and all equipment, including an emergency resuscitation cart (or trolley). Many units also have fully equipped mobile carts to travel to other sites when needed, preferably in a designated storage area near the procedure rooms to avoid obstructing the hallways, as required by regulations.

Staff

Specially trained endoscopy assistants have many important functions. They:
- *prepare patients* for their procedures, physically and mentally;
- *set up* all necessary equipment;
- *assist* endoscopists during procedures;
- *monitor* patients' safety, sedation, and recovery;
- *clean*, disinfect, and process equipment;
- *maintain quality control*.

Most endoscopy assistants are trained nurses, but technicians and nursing aides also have roles (e.g. in equipment processing). Large units need a variety of other staff, to handle reception, transport, reporting, and equipment management, including informatics.

Members of staff need places to change, store their clothes and valuables, and a break area for refreshments and meals.

Procedure reports

There are three broad areas of procedural documentation: nursing documentation before, during, and after the procedure, the endoscopy report, and a sedation record if a separate provider administers sedation. Space and workstations in the room are essential to maintain efficiency for the endoscopist and supporting team members.

Nursing record

The nurse's report usually takes the form of a preprinted "flow sheet," with places to record all of the pre-procedure safety checks, personnel present, vital signs, use of sedation/analgesia and other medications, monitoring of vital signs and patient responses, equipment and accessory usage, and image documentation. It concludes with post-sedation monitoring, documentation of the requirements for discharge, and discharge instructions given to the patient.

Procedure report

In many units, the endoscopist's report is generated in the procedure rooms. In larger ones, there may need to be a separate work area designed for this purpose.

The report includes the patient's demographics, reasons for the procedure (indications), specific medical risks and precautions, sedation/analgesia, findings, specimens, treatments, conclusions, follow-up plans, and any adverse events. Endoscopists use many reporting methods—handwritten notes, preprinted forms, free dictation, and electronic endoscopy reporting systems. Recommended endoscopy reporting elements have been set out by endoscopy-related societies, including the World Endoscopy Organization, the American Society for Gastrointestinal Endoscopy (ASGE), the Canadian Association of Gastroenterology, the

European Society of Gastrointestinal Endoscopy, and the North American and European Societies of Pediatric Gastroenterology, Hepatology and Nutrition.

The paperless endoscopy unit

In many units nowadays, all reporting and photo-documentation (nursing, administrative, and endoscopic) is incorporated into a comprehensive electronic endoscopy reporting system. Such systems substantially reduce the paperwork burden, facilitate standardized documentation, enable integration of histopathology, allow tracking and tracing of equipment, and increase both efficiency and quality assurance.

Management, behavior, and teamwork

Complex organizations require efficient management and leadership. This works best as a collaborative exercise between the medical director of endoscopy and the chief nurse or endoscopy nurse manager. The biggest units will also have a separate administrator. These individuals must be skilled in handling people (endoscopists, staff, and patients), complex equipment, and significant financial resources. They must develop and maintain good working relationships with many departments within the hospital (such as radiology, pathology, sterile processing, infection control, anesthesia, bioengineering), as well as numerous manufacturers and vendors. They also need to be fully cognizant of all of the many local and national regulations that now impact on endoscopic practice.

The wise endoscopist will embrace the team approach, and realize that maintaining an atmosphere of collegiality and mutual respect is essential for efficiency, job satisfaction, and staff retention, and for optimal patient outcomes.

It is also essential to ensure that the push for efficiency does not drive out humanity. Patients should not be packaged as mere commodities during the endoscopy process. Treating our patients (and those who accompany them) with respect and courtesy is fundamental. Always assume that patients are listening, even if they are apparently sedated, so never chatter about irrelevances in their presence. Maintain infection control practices and never eat or drink in patient areas. Background music is appreciated by many patients and staff but may potentially cognitively overload more novice endoscopists.

Documentation and quality improvement

The agreed policies of the unit (including regulations dictated by the hospital and national organizations) are enshrined in an *Endoscopy Unit Procedure Manual*. This must be easily available, constantly updated, and frequently consulted.

Day-to-day documentation includes details of staff and room usage, disinfection processes, medications, instrument and accessory use, as well as the procedure reports.

A formal quality assessment and improvement process is essential for maximizing the quality, safety and efficiency of endoscopy services. Professional societies have recommended methods and metrics for units to assess or demonstrate whether the services they provide are patient-centered, safe, high-quality, and appropriate. The ASGE has incorporated these into its Endoscopy Unit Recognition Program, and the benefit of concentrating on and documenting quality is well exemplified by the success of the endoscopy Global Rating Scale as a patient-centered quality improvement tool in the United Kingdom and Canada.

The Society of Gastroenterology Nurses and Associates (SGNA) in the United States has an Infection Prevention Champion Program to guide units on ways of improving quality and helps to ensure that most current and safe practices are followed. SGNA recognizes endoscopy units that have shown a commitment to infection prevention, a supportive and educational work environment and positive patient outcomes through the Flame Award for Unit Excellence.

Educational resources

Endoscopy units should offer educational resources for all of its users, including patients, staff, and endoscopists. Clinical staff need a selection of relevant books, atlases, journals, and publications of professional societies. Many organizations also produce useful educational videos. Increasingly, many of these materials are available online, so easy internet access is essential.

Teaching units should embrace endoscopy simulators, which are valuable tools for training and assessment. Units should have dedicated time for education, and regular staff meetings.

Further reading

Armstrong D, Barkun A, Bridges R, et al. Canadian Association of Gastroenterology consensus guidelines on safety and quality indicators in endoscopy. *Can J Gastroenterol* 2012;26(1):17–31.

Bretthauer M, Aabakken L, Dekker E, et al. Reporting systems in gastrointestinal endoscopy: Requirements and standards facilitating quality improvement: European Society of Gastrointestinal Endoscopy position statement. *United Eur Gastroenterol J* 2016;4(1):172–6.

Cotton PB, Eisen GM, Aabakken L, et al. A lexicon for endoscopic adverse events: Report of an ASGE workshop. *Gastrointest Endosc* 2010;71(3):446–54.

Day LW, Muthusamy VR, Collins, J, et al. Multisociety guideline on reprocessing flexible GI endoscopes and accessories. *Gastrointest Endosc* 2021;93(1):11–33.

Hitchins CR, Metzner M, Edworthy J, et al. Non-technical skills and gastrointestinal endoscopy: A review of the literature. *Frontline Gastroenterol* 2018;9(2):129–34.

Joint Advisory Group on Gastrointestinal Endoscopy (JAG). Global Rating Scale (GRS) version for non-acute services (all nations). London, United Kingdom, 2016. Available at: www.thejag.org.uk.

Lightdale JR, Walsh CM, Narula CM, et al. Pediatric Endoscopy Quality Improvement Network quality standards and indicators for pediatric endoscopy facilities: A joint NASPGHAN/ESPGHAN guideline. *J Pediatr Gastroenterol Nutr* 2022;74(S1 Suppl 1):S16–S29.

Marques S, Bispo M, Pimentel-Nunes P, et al. Image documentation in gastrointestinal endoscopy: Review of recommendations. *GE Port J Gastroenterol* 2017;24(6):269–74.

Mulder JJ, Jacobs MAJM, Leicester RJ, et al. Guidelines for designing a digestive disease endoscopy unit: Report of the World Endoscopy Organization. *Dig Endos* 2013;25(4):365–75.

Narula P, Broughton R, Howarth L, et al. Paediatric endoscopy Global Rating Scale: Development of a quality improvement tool and results of a national pilot. *J Pediatr Gastroenterol Nutr* 2019;69(2):171–5.

Pall H, Lerner D, Khlevner J, et al. Developing the pediatric gastrointestinal endoscopy unit: A clinical report by the Endoscopy and Procedures Committee. *J Pediatr Gastroenterol Nutr* 2016;63(2):295–306.

Rees CJ, Thomas Gibson S, Rutter MD, et al. British Society of Gastroenterology, the Joint Advisory Group on GI Endoscopy, the Association of Coloproctology of Great Britain and Ireland. UK key performance indicators and quality assurance standards for colonoscopy. *Gut* 2016;65(12):1923–9.

Rizk MK, Sawhney MS, Cohen J, et al. Quality indicators common to all GI endoscopic procedures. *Am J Gastroenterol* 2015;110(1):48–59.

Sultan S, Lim JK, Altayar O, et al. AGA rapid recommendations for gastrointestinal procedures during the COVID-19 pandemic. *Gastroenterology* 2020;159(2):739–58.

Valori, RM, Johnston DJ. Leadership and team building in gastrointestinal endoscopy. *Best Pract Res Clin Gastroenterol* 2016;30(3):497–509.

Walsh CM, Lightdale JR, Mack DR, et al. Overview of the Pediatric Endoscopy Quality Improvement Network quality standards and indicators for pediatric endoscopy: A joint NASPGHAN/ESPGHAN guideline. *J Pediatr Gastroenterol Nutr* 2022;74(S1 Suppl 1):S3–S15.

CHAPTER 3
Endoscopic Equipment

Endoscopes

There are many different endoscopes available for various applications, and several manufacturers of them, but they all have common features. There is a control head with valves (buttons) for CO_2/air insufflation and suction, a flexible shaft (insertion tube) carrying the light guide and one or more service channels, and a maneuverable bending section at the tip. An umbilical or universal cord (also called "light guide connecting tube") connects the endoscope to the light source and processor, CO_2/air supply, and suction (Fig 3.1). Illumination is provided from an external high-intensity source through one or more light-carrying fiber bundles.

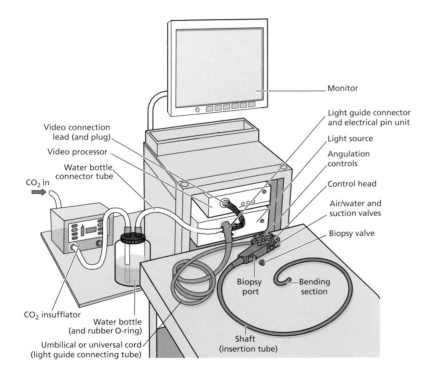

Fig 3.1 Endoscope system.

Cotton and Williams' Practical Gastrointestinal Endoscopy: The Fundamentals, Eighth Edition.
Catharine M. Walsh, Ahmir Ahmad, Brian P. Saunders, Jonathan Cohen, Peter B. Cotton, and Christopher B. Williams.
© 2024 John Wiley & Sons Ltd. Published 2024 by John Wiley & Sons Ltd.
Companion website: www.wiley.com/go/cottonwilliams8e

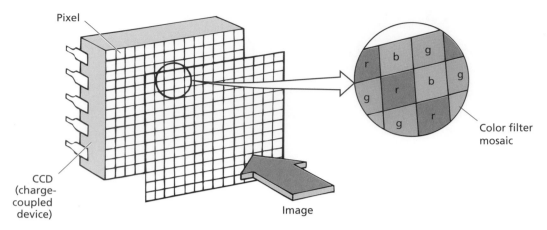

Fig 3.2 Static red, green, and blue filters in the "color" chip.

The image is captured with a charge-coupled device (CCD) chip, transmitted electronically, and displayed on a video monitor. Individual pixels (photocells) in the CCD chips can respond only to degrees of light and dark. Color appreciation is arranged by two methods. So-called "color CCDs" have their pixels arranged under a series of color filter stripes (Fig 3.2). By contrast, "monochrome CCDs" (or, more correctly, sequential system CCDs) use a rotating color filter wheel to illuminate all of the pixels with primary color strobe-effect lighting (Fig 3.3). This type of chip can be made smaller, or can give higher resolution, but the system is more expensive because of the additional mechanics and image-processing technology. Progress has also been made in magnifying

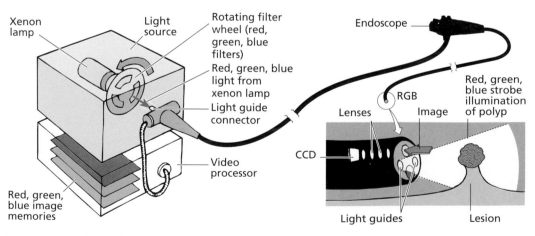

Fig 3.3 Sequential color illumination.

endoscopic images. High-magnification endoscopes have an optical zoom, generated by a movable lens in the endoscope tip, which maintains the image display quality. Alternatively, electronic, or digital magnification enlarges the image but decreases image quality. Most available endoscopes have combined optical and digital zoom, while some have near-focus imaging that allows the endoscope to be moved closer (within 2–6 mm) to an area of interest while still maintaining focus.

"Electronic chromoendoscopy" systems are now standard in many endoscopes, allowing enhancement of aspects of the surface of the gastrointestinal mucosa. Narrow band imaging (NBI; Olympus Corporation) uses optical filters to select certain wavelengths of light, which correspond to the peak light absorption of hemoglobin, enhancing the visualization of blood vessels and certain surface structures. The Fuji Intelligent Chromo Endoscopy (FICE; Fujinon Endoscopy) and i-Scan (Pentax Medical) systems take ordinary endoscopic images and digitally process the output to estimate different wavelengths of light, providing a number of different imaging outputs. Autofluorescence imaging can detect endogenous fluorophores, a number of which occur in the gastrointestinal tract. Two systems now also allow magnification of the endoscopic image down to the cellular level: termed confocal laser endomicroscopy (Pentax Medical, Mauna Kea Technologies). Blue laser light is focused on the desired tissue after injecting fluorescent materials which become excited by the laser light and are detected by the confocal optical unit at defined horizontal levels.

Tip control

The distal bending section (10 cm or so) and tip of the endoscope are fully deflectable, usually in both planes, up to 180° or more. Control depends upon pull wires attached at the tip just beneath the outer protective sheath and passing back through the length of the instrument shaft to the two angulation control knobs or dials on the control head (Fig 3.4). The larger knob deflects the tip up and down, whereas the smaller one is responsible for lateral control (i.e. right or left). The knobs incorporate a friction braking system, so that the tip can be fixed temporarily in any desired position. Some ultra-thin endoscopes only have a single dial for up/down tip deflection and require application of torque for sideways maneuverability. The instrument shaft is torque stable, so that rotating movements applied to the head are transmitted to the tip when the shaft is relatively straight. Some colonoscopes incorporate a variable-stiffness function, controlled by a rotatable dial on the control head, which enables stiffening of the insertion tube beyond 30 cm from the instrument tip, so the distal portion remains easily deflectable. Duodenoscopes used for endoscopic retrograde cholangiopancreatography (ERCP) and linear echoendoscopes have an additional dial for controlling the elevator.

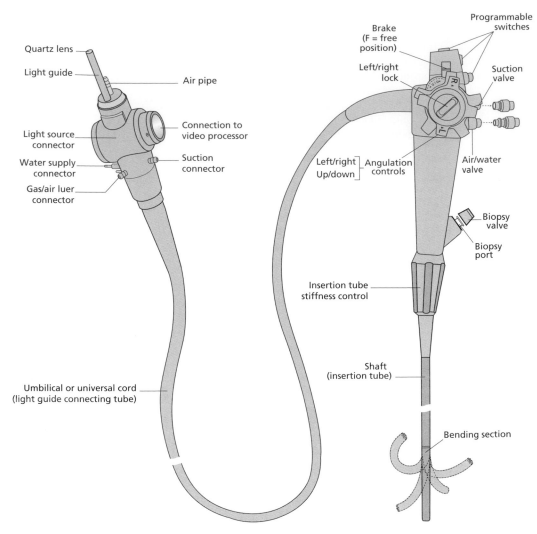

Quartz lens

Light guide

Air pipe

Light source connector

Connection to video processor

Water supply connector

Suction connector

Gas/air luer connector

Brake (F = free position)

Programmable switches

Left/right lock

Suction valve

Left/right Up/down

Angulation controls

Air/water valve

Biopsy valve

Biopsy port

Insertion tube stiffness control

Umbilical or universal cord (light guide connecting tube)

Shaft (insertion tube)

Bending section

Fig 3.4 Basic design of the endoscope.

Instrument channels and valves

The internal anatomy of endoscopes is complex (Fig 3.5). The shaft incorporates a biopsy/suction or "working channel" extending from the entry "biopsy port" to the tip of the instrument to enable passage of endoscopic accessories, such as biopsy forceps, probes, and snares, through the length of the endoscope (Fig 3.6). The channel is usually about 3 mm in diameter but varies from 1 to 5 mm depending upon the purpose for which the endoscope was designed (from neonatal examinations to major therapeutic procedures). In some instruments, especially those with lateral-viewing optics, the tip of the channel incorporates a deflectable elevator or bridge (Fig 3.7), which permits directional control of forceps and other accessories independent of the instrument tip. This elevator is controlled by an additional thumb lever on the control head. The working channel is also

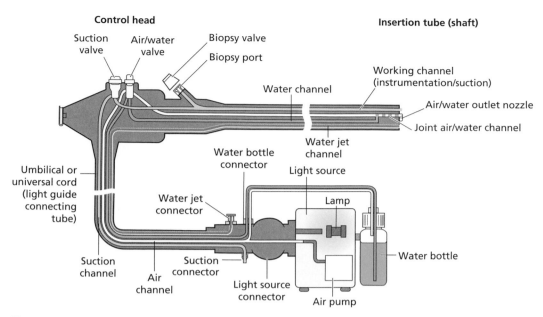

Fig 3.5 The internal anatomy of a typical endoscope.

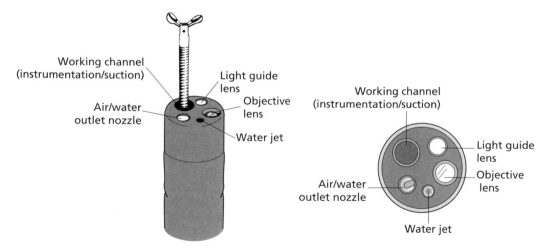

Fig 3.6 The tip of a forward-viewing endoscope.

involved in the application of suction to aspirate secretions: an external suction pump is connected to the universal cord near to the light source, and suction is diverted into the instrument channel by pressing the suction valve on the control head. Another small channel allows the passage of CO_2/air to distend the organ being examined. The CO_2/air is supplied from a pump in the light source and insufflation is controlled by covering the vent hole on the air/water valve. For colonoscopy, the insufflation system can be modified to CO_2 rather than room air and has been shown to lessen abdominal distension and pain after colonoscopy. The CO_2/air system also pressurizes the water bottle, so that a jet of water can be squirted across the distal lens to clean it when the air/water valve is depressed.

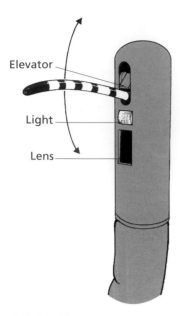

Fig 3.7 A side-viewing endoscope with a deflectable elevator.

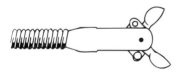

Fig 3.8 Biopsy cups open.

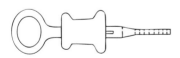

Fig 3.9 Control handle for biopsy forceps.

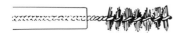

Fig 3.10 Cytology brush with outer sleeve.

Different instruments

The endoscopy unit must have a selection of endoscopes for specific applications. These may differ in length, size, stiffness, channel size and number, sophistication, and distal lens orientation. Most endoscopies are performed with instruments providing *direct forward vision*, via a wide-angle lens (up to 130°) (Fig 3.6). However, there are circumstances in which it is preferable to view *laterally*, particularly for endoscopic retrograde cholangiopancreatography (ERCP) (Fig 3.7). An understanding of the spatial orientation of the various ports and components of endoscopes is important, especially in planning complex therapeutic interventions.

The overall diameter of an endoscope is a compromise between engineering ideals and patient tolerance. The shaft must contain and protect many bundles, wires, and tubes, all of which are stronger and more efficient when larger (Fig 3.5). A colonoscope can reasonably approach 15 mm in diameter, but this size is acceptable in the upper gut only for specialized therapeutic instruments.

Routine upper endoscopy is mostly performed with instruments of 8–11 mm diameter. Smaller endoscopes are available; they are better tolerated by all patients and have specific application in children. Some can be passed through the nose rather than the mouth. However, smaller instruments inevitably involve some compromise in durability, image quality, maneuverability, biopsy size, and therapeutic potential.

Several companies now produce a full range of endoscopes at comparable prices. However, light sources and processors produced by different companies are not interchangeable, so that most endoscopy units concentrate for convenience on equipment from a single manufacturer. Endoscopes are delicate, and some breakages are inevitable. Careful maintenance and close communication, repair, and back-up arrangements with an efficient company are necessary to maintain an endoscopy service. The quality of that support is often a crucial factor affecting the choice of company.

Endoscopic accessories

Many devices can be passed through the endoscope working channel for diagnostic and therapeutic purposes.
- *Biopsy forceps* consist of a pair of sharpened cups (Fig 3.8), a spiral metal cable, a pull wire, and a control handle (Fig 3.9). Their maximum diameter is limited by the size of the channel, and the length of the cups by the radius of curvature through which they must pass in the instrument tip. When taking biopsy specimens from a lesion that can only be approached tangentially (e.g. the wall of the esophagus), forceps with a central spike may be helpful; however, these do present a significant puncture hazard for staff.
- *Cytology brushes* have a covering plastic sleeve to protect the specimen during withdrawal (Fig 3.10).
- *Flexible needles* are used for injections and for sampling fluids and cells.
- *Fluid-flushing devices*. Many instruments have an auxiliary water ("water jet") channel that can be connected to an external high-flow irrigation pump to produce a forward-directed water

spray from the tip of the endoscope, which can be useful for cleaning the lens and mucosa as well as water immersion or exchange (see Chapter 7). This is usually controlled by a foot switch or remote control. Fluids can also be forcibly flushed through the instrumentation channel with a large syringe or a pulsatile electric pump, with a suitable nozzle inserted into the biopsy port. For more precise aiming, a washing catheter can be passed down the channel to clean specific areas of interest, or to highlight mucosal detail by "dye spraying" (using a nozzle-tipped catheter).

Ancillary equipment

- *Suction traps* (fitted temporarily into the suction line) can be used to take samples of intestinal secretions and bile for microbiology, chemistry, and cytology (Fig 3.11; see also Figs 8.7 and 8.8).
- *Biteguards* are used to protect the patient's teeth and the endoscope. Some guards have straps, to keep them in place, and oxygen ports.
- *Overtubes* are flexible plastic sleeves that cover the endoscope shaft and act as a conduit for repeated intubations, or to facilitate therapeutic procedures such as the extraction of a foreign body and hemostasis (Fig 3.12).

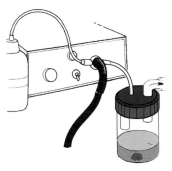

Fig 3.11 A suction trap to collect fluid specimens.

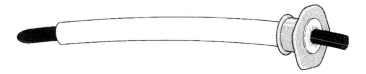

Fig 3.12 An overtube with biteguard over a rubber lavage tube.

- *Caps* of various shapes can be attached to the tip of the endoscope to facilitate various procedures, such as banding and mucosal resection, and dissection (Fig 7.6).
- *Stretchers/trolleys*. Endoscopy is normally performed on a standard transportation stretcher. This should have side rails, and preferably allow height adjustment. The ability to tilt the stretcher head down may be helpful in emergencies.
- *Image documentation*. Videoscopes capture images digitally, which can then be enhanced, stored, transmitted, and printed. Video sequences can also be recorded digitally.
- *Sedation and monitoring*. All patients require regular monitoring during an endoscopy with pulse oximetry as a minimum. For patients undergoing moderate ("conscious") or deep sedation, recommended minimal patient monitoring includes non-invasive assessment of blood pressure, heart rate, pulse oximetry and visual assessment of ventilatory activity, level of consciousness, and discomfort. Continuous electrocardiogram (ECG) monitoring is generally recommended during long procedures and for patients at high risk, including the elderly and patients with significant cardiovascular or pulmonary disease or a history of dysrhythmias. Many units also have the facility for end tidal CO_2 monitoring, particularly for deeply sedated patients. Appropriate resuscitation equipment must be available, including oral airways, oxygen delivery systems, and wall suction. Endoscopy facilities where pediatric procedures are performed should ensure availability of pediatric-specific monitoring and resuscitation equipment.

Electrosurgical units

Any electrosurgical unit can be used for endoscopic therapy, if necessary, but purpose-built isolated-circuit and "intelligent" units have major advantages in safety and ease of use. Units should have test circuitry and an automatic warning system or cut-out in case a connection is faulty or the patient plate is not in contact. Most units have separate "cut" and "coagulate" circuits, which can often be blended to choice. For flexible endoscopy, low-power settings are used (typically 15–50 W). However, an "auto-cut" option is increasingly popular. This uses an apparently higher power setting but gives good control of tissue heating and cutting, because the system automatically adjusts power output according to initial tissue resistance and increasing resistance during coagulation and desiccation.

The type of current is generally less important than the amount of power produced, and other physical factors such as electrode pressure or snare-wire thickness and squeeze are more critical. High settings (high power) of coagulating current provide satisfactory cutting characteristics, whereas units with output not rated directly in watts can be assumed to have "cut" power output much greater than that of "coag" at the same setting. The difference in current type used is therefore often illusory. If in doubt, pure coagulating current alone is considered by most expert endoscopists to be safer and more predictable, giving a "slow cook" effect and maximum hemostasis. Principles of electrosurgery are outlined further in Chapter 8.

Lasers and argon plasma coagulation

Lasers (particularly the neodymium-YAG and argon lasers) were introduced into endoscopy for treatment of bleeding ulcers and for tumor ablation, because it seemed desirable to use a "no touch" technique. However, it has become clear that the same effects can be achieved with simpler devices, and that pressure (coaptation) may actually help hemostasis.

Argon plasma coagulation (*APC*) is easier to use and as effective as lasers for most endoscopic purposes. APC electrocoagulates, without tissue contact, by using the electrical conductivity of argon gas—a similar phenomenon to that seen in neon lights. The argon, passed down an electrode catheter (Fig 3.13a) and energized with an intelligent-circuitry electrosurgical unit and patient plate, ionizes to produce a local plasma arc—like a miniature lightning strike (Fig 3.13b). The heating effect is inherently superficial (2–3 mm at most, unless current is applied in the same place for many seconds), because tissue coagulation increases resistance and causes the plasma arc to jump elsewhere. For coagulation, compared with contact techniques, APC provides a more homogeneous tissue effect and can treat large surface areas more rapidly. However, it lacks the mechanical tamponade hemostatic effect of contact methods. It is mainly used for coagulating superficial vascular lesions, palliative ablation of tumors, and ablation of residual polyp tissue after piecemeal snare-loop removal of a large polyp, as it is too superficial to debulk a large lesion primarily. However, combined submucosal injection of a microjet of saline cushion with higher-watt APC

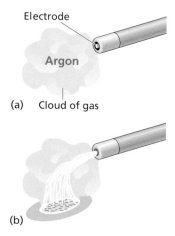

Electrode

Argon

(a)   Cloud of gas

(b)

Fig 3.13 Argon plasma coagulation (APC).

ablation, so-called "hybrid-APC," has been applied to achieve controlled complete ablation of tissue to the submucosa.

Equipment maintenance

Endoscopes are expensive and complex tools. They should be stored safely, hanging vertically in cupboards through which air can circulate. Care must be taken when carrying instruments, as the optics are easily damaged if left to dangle or are knocked against a hard surface. The control head, tip, and umbilical cord should all be held (Fig 3.14).

The life of an endoscope is largely determined by the quality of maintenance. Complex accessories (e.g. electrosurgical equipment) must be checked and kept in safe condition. Close collaboration with hospital bioengineering departments and servicing engineers is essential. Repairs and maintenance must be properly documented.

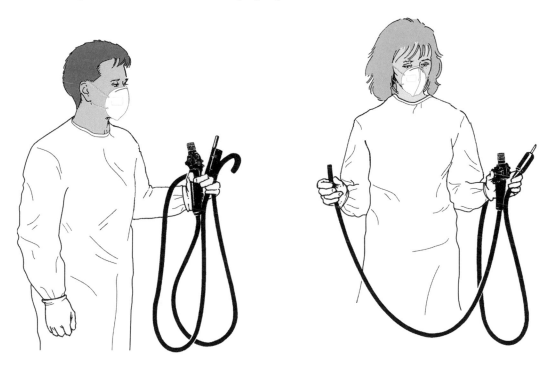

Fig 3.14 Carry endoscopes carefully to avoid knocks to the optics in the control head and tip.

Channel blockage

Blockage of the air/water (or biopsy/suction) channel is one of the most common endoscope problems. Special channel-flushing devices are available, allowing separate syringe flushing of the air and water channels; they should be used routinely. When blockage occurs, the various systems and connections (instrument umbilical, water bottle cap or tube, etc.) must be checked, including the tightness and the presence of rubber O-rings where relevant. It is usually possible to clear the different channels by using the manufacturer's flushing device or a syringe with a suitable soft plastic introducer or micropipette tip. Water can be injected down any channel and, because water is not compressed, more force can be applied than with air. Remember that a small syringe (1–5 mL) generates more pressure than a large one, whereas a large one (50 mL) generates more suction. The air or suction connections at the umbilical, or the water tube within the water bottle, can be syringed until water emerges from the instrument tip. Care should be taken to cover or depress the relevant control valves while syringing. Another method for unclogging the suction channel is to remove the valve and apply suction directly at the port.

Infection control

There is a risk of transmitting infection in the endoscopy unit from patient to patient, patient to staff, and even from staff to patient. Universal precautions should always be adopted. This means assuming that all patients are infectious, even if there is no objective evidence. Infection control experts and equipment manufacturers should be welcomed as partners in minimizing infection risk; they should be invited to participate in developing unit policies and in monitoring their effectiveness through formal quality control processes. Infection control policies should be written down and understood by all staff.

Staff protection

Staff should be immunized against hepatitis and severe acute res-piratory syndrome coronavirus 2 (SARS-CoV-2); tuberculosis checks are mandatory in some units. Splashing with body fluids is a risk for staff in contact with patients and instruments. Additionally, endoscopy is considered an aerosol-generating procedure (as is intubation) with the potential for transmission of airborne viruses. Masks (surgical or N95/N99 respirator, depending on local guid-ance), long-sleeved fluid-repellent gowns, gloves, and face shields or eye protection should be worn for these activities (Fig 3.15).

Other measures to reduce the risk of infection include:
- *frequent hand-washing*;
- *use of paper towels* when handling soiled accessories;
- disposal of *soiled items* directly into a sink or designated area (not on clean surfaces);
- *separate disposal of hazardous waste*, needles, and syringes;
- *covering skin breaks* with a waterproof dressing;
- *maintenance of good hygienic practice* throughout the unit.

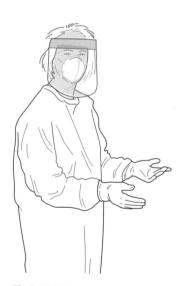

Fig 3.15 Mask, gowns, gloves, and eye/face protection should be worn.

Cleaning and disinfection

There are three levels of disinfection:

1 *Low- or intermediate-level disinfection* (essentially "wipe-down") is adequate for *non-critical devices*, which do not come into contact with the patient or touch only intact skin, such as blood pressure cuffs, cameras, and endoscopic furniture.

2 *High-level disinfection* or, if possible, *sterilization* is required for *semi-critical devices* which come into contact with mucous mem-branes or nonintact skin and do not penetrate sterile tissue. These include endoscopes and esophageal dilators.

3 *Sterilization* (destruction of all microbial life) is required for ***critical devices*** that enter the vascular system or sterile tissue, including endoscopes used in sterile settings and endoscopic equipment used for invasive procedures such as ERCP and endoscopic ultrasound, and equipment such as biopsy forceps, sclerotherapy needles, and sphincterotomes. "Single-use" disposable items are pre-sterilized.

Endoscope reprocessing

Guidelines for cleaning and disinfecting endoscopes should be determined in each unit (and documented in the procedure manual) after consulting with manufacturers, infection control experts, and appropriate national advisory bodies. Endoscopists should be fully aware of their local practice, not least because they may be held legally responsible for any untoward event. All advisory bodies require high-level disinfection of endoscopes and other equipment shortly after use. There is no need for specific alterations in reprocessing protocols for SARS-CoV-2 given that the viricidal nature of detergents used in reprocessing are effective at inactivating coronaviruses.

How long a disinfected instrument remains fit for use after disinfection is an important issue, and still a matter for debate. Some authorities have recommended 4–7 days, but the reality depends on several factors. Endoscopes that contain retained moisture will rapidly become colonized by the rinsing water. Assiduous care must be taken in the drying process, and specially designed drying cabinets are available commercially. Local policy should be guided by national recommendations and can be validated by microbiological monitoring.

Formal cleaning and disinfection procedures should take place in a purpose-designed area. There should be clearly defined and separate clean and dirty areas, multiple worktops, and double sinks as well as a separate hand washbasin, endoscopic reprocessors (washing machines), and ultrasonic cleaners. An appropriately placed fume hood is also desirable. When cleaning endoscopes, individuals should wear appropriate personal protective equipment, including fluid-repellent gowns, gloves, and eye/face protection.

Mechanical cleaning

The first and vitally important task in the disinfection process is to clean the endoscope and all of its channels, to remove all blood, secretions, and debris. Disinfectants cannot penetrate organic material.

Initial cleaning must be done immediately after the endoscope is removed from the patient and prior to disconnecting the endoscope from the power source.

1 *Wipe down* the insertion tube and distal end with a cloth soaked in enzymatic detergent.

2 *Suck water and enzymatic detergent* through the working (suction/biopsy) channel, alternating with air, until the solution is visibly clean.

3 *Flush the air/water channel* with the manufacturer's flushing device or by depressing the air/water button while occluding the water bottle attachment at the light source and holding the tip of the scope under water. This should be continued until vigorous bubbling is seen.

4 *Flush the auxiliary-water channel and elevator-wire channel* (if applicable) using a syringe or irrigation pump to ensure there is no blockage.

5 *Detach the endoscope* from the light source and suction pump.

6 *Attach the cap that protects the electrical connections* and transfer the scope (in protective packaging to avoid contamination) to the designated cleaning area.

7 *Remove all valves and biopsy caps.*

8 *Test the scope for leaks*, particularly in the bending section, by pressurizing it with the leak-testing device and immersing the instrument in water. Angulate the bending section in its four directions while the instrument is under pressure to identify leaks in the distal rubber that are only obvious when it is stretched. Ensure that all pressure is removed before disconnecting the leak tester.

9 *Totally immerse the instrument* in warm water and neutral detergent, and then wash the outside of the instrument thoroughly with a soft cloth.

10 *Brush the distal end* with a soft brush while immersed, paying particular attention to the air/water outlet jet and any bridge/elevator.

11 *Clean the biopsy/suction channel opening and suction port*, while immersed, using the port-cleaning brush provided. Pass a clean channel-cleaning brush suitable for the instrument and channel size through the biopsy/suction channel until it emerges clean (at least three times), cleaning the brush itself each time before reinsertion. Pass the cleaning brush from the biopsy/suction channel opening in the other direction.

12 *Place the endoscope into a reprocessor* to complete cleaning and disinfection (or continue manually).

13 *Clean all instrument accessories* equally scrupulously, including the air/water and suction valves, auxiliary-water/elevator-wire channel, water bottles, and cleaning brushes.

Manual cleaning

After brushing:

1 *Attach the manufacturer's cleaning adapters* to the biopsy/suction, air/water, and auxiliary-water/elevator-wire channels. Ensure that the instrument remains immersed in the detergent fluid.

2 *Flush each channel with detergent* fluid, ensuring that it emerges from the distal end of each channel.

3 *Leave in detergent* for the time stated by the manufacturer of the detergent product used.

4 *Purge detergent from the channels.*

5 *Flush each channel with clean water* to rinse the detergent fluid.

6 *Rinse the exterior of the endoscope.*

7 *Check that all air is expelled from the channels.*

Manual disinfection

Soak the instrument and accessories (such as valves) in the chosen disinfectant for the recommended contact time.

Disinfectants

Glutaraldehyde has been the most popular agent. It can destroy viruses and bacteria within a few minutes, is non-corrosive (to endoscopes), and has a low surface tension, which aids penetration.

The length of contact time needed for disinfection varies according to the type of glutaraldehyde used, and the temperature. Guidelines vary between countries, but 20 minutes is commonly recommended. More prolonged soaking may be required in cases of known or suspected mycobacterial disease.

Glutaraldehyde does carry the risk of sensitization, and can cause severe dermatitis, sinusitis, or asthma among exposed staff. The risk increases with increasing levels and duration of exposure. Medical-grade latex gloves, or nitrile rubber gloves, should be worn, with goggles and/or a face mask to protect against splashes. Closed system reprocessors and fume hoods/extraction fans are important. Reprocessors should be self-disinfecting. The concentration of disinfectant should be monitored.

Peracetic acid, chlorine dioxide, Sterox, and other agents have also been used for endoscope disinfection.

A *sterile water supply* (special filters may be needed) helps to reduce the risk of nosocomial infections.

Rinsing, drying, and storing

Following disinfection, reprocessors rinse the instruments internally and externally to remove all traces of disinfectant, using the all-channel irrigator. The exterior should be completely dried using a clean, lint-free cloth. The air, water, and biopsy/suction channels (and flushing and forceps elevation channels if fitted) are perfused with 70% alcohol and dried with forced air before storage. This must be done for all endoscopes processed either manually or by automated reprocessor (some reprocessors have this function as part of the cycle). Bacteria multiply in a moist environment, and the importance of drying instruments after disinfection cannot be overemphasized. Instruments should be hung vertically in a well-ventilated, dust-free cupboard.

Accessory devices

Diagnostic and therapeutic devices (such as biopsy forceps) are critical accessories and must be sterile. Many are now disposable. Reusable accessories, such as water bottles, are autoclaved or gas sterilized.

Quality control of reprocessing

All institutional processes and quality monitors used during endoscope reprocessing should be documented. Records should also be kept of the disinfection process for every endoscope, including who cleaned it, when, and how. Records that link the endoscope with which the patient was examined should also be kept. Routine microbiological surveillance of automatic disinfectors and endoscopes is recommended by some experts but is not endorsed by many of the main national societies, and is not widely practiced. This should allow early detection of serious contaminating organisms such as *Pseudomonas* and atypical mycobacteria. Routine surveillance also allows the early detection of otherwise unrecognizable internal channel damage and reprocessing protocol errors, as well as any water and environmental contamination problems. The specter of prion-related disease may be raised in patients with degenerative neurological symptoms. As prion proteins are not inactivated by heat or current disinfection regimes, disposable accessories should be used with a back-up endoscope reserved for such suspect patients.

Remember, although most of the cleaning, disinfection, and maintenance activities are normally and appropriately delegated to the staff, it is the endoscopist who is responsible for ensuring that their equipment is safe to use. Endoscopists should know how to complete the process themselves, especially in some emergency situations where the usual endoscopy nurses may not be available.

Further reading

ASGE Standards of Practice Committee, Early DS, Lightdale JR, et al. Guidelines for sedation and anesthesia in GI endoscopy. *Gastrointest Endosc* 2018;87(2):327–37.

ASGE Technology Committee, Komanduri S, Dayyeh BKA, et al. Technologies for monitoring the quality of endoscope reprocessing. *Gastrointest Endosc* 2014;80(3):369–73.

ASGE Technology Committee, Lo SK, Fujii-Lau LL, et al. The use of carbon dioxide in gastrointestinal endoscopy. *Gastrointest Endosc* 2016;83(5):857–65.

ASGE Technology Committee, Parsi MA, Sullivan SA, et al. Automated endoscope reprocessors. *Gastrointest Endosc* 2016;84(6):885–92.

Allison MC, Bradley CR, Griffiths H, et al. BSG guidance for decontamination of equipment for gastrointestinal endoscopy. Available at: www.bsg.org.uk/resource-type/clinical-resources/guidance.

Beilenhoff U, Biering H, Blum R, et al. Reprocessing of flexible endoscopes and endoscopic accessories used in gastrointestinal endoscopy: Position Statement of the European Society of Gastrointestinal Endoscopy (ESGE) and European Society of Gastroenterology Nurses and Associates (ESGENA)—Update 2018. *Endoscopy* 2018;50(12):1205–34.

Beilenhoff U, Biering H, Blum R, et al. Prevention of multidrug-resistant infections from contaminated duodenoscopes: Position Statement of the European Society of Gastrointestinal Endoscopy (ESGE) and European Society of Gastroenterology Nurses and Associates (ESGENA). *Endoscopy* 2017;49(11):1098–106.

Day LW, Muthusamy VR, Collins JR, et al. Multisociety guideline on reprocessing flexible GI endoscopes and accessories. *Gastrointest Endosc* 2021;93(1):11–33.

Dossa F, Megetto O, Yakubu, et al. Sedation practices for routine gastrointestinal endoscopy: A systematic review of recommendations. *BMC Gastroenterol* 2021:7;21(1):22.

Rey JF, Beilenhoff U, Neumann CS, et al. European Society of Gastrointestinal Endoscopy (ESGE) guideline: The use of electrosurgical units. *Endoscopy* 2010;42(9):764–72.

Trindade AJ, Copland A, Bhatt, et al. Single-use duodenoscopes and duodenoscopes with disposable end caps. *Gastrointest Endosc* 2021; 93(5):997–1005.

CHAPTER 4

Patient Care, Risks, and Safety

Skilled endoscopists can now reach every part of the digestive tract and its appendages, such as the biliary tree and pancreas. It is possible to take specimens from all of these areas, and to treat many of their afflictions, so patients have benefited greatly from endoscopy. Unfortunately, however, in some cases the procedure may not be helpful, and can even result in severe adverse events. There are also some hazards for the staff. The goal must be to maximize the benefits and minimize the risks. We need competent endoscopists, performing procedures for proper indications on patients who are fully educated and prepared, with skilled assistants, and using optimum equipment. The basic principles are similar for all areas of gastrointestinal endoscopy, recognizing that there are specific circumstances where the risks are greater, including therapeutic and emergency procedures.

Patient assessment

Endoscopy is normally part of a comprehensive evaluation by a gastroenterologist or other digestive specialist. It is mostly used electively in the practice environment or hospital outpatient clinic, but sometimes may be needed in any part of a healthcare facility (e.g. emergency room, intensive care unit, operating room). Sometimes endoscopists offer an "open access" service, where the initial clinical assessment and continuing care are performed by another physician. In all of these situations it is the responsibility of the endoscopist to ensure that the potential benefits exceed the potential risks, and to personally perform the necessary evaluations to make appropriate recommendations for the patient.

Is the procedure indicated?
Gastrointestinal endoscopy is a primary tool for evaluating the esophagus, stomach, small and large intestines. It may be used for many reasons. Broadly speaking, the goal may be to:
1 *make a diagnosis* in the presence of suggestive symptoms (e.g. dyspepsia, dysphagia, anorexia, weight loss, diarrhea, anemia);
2 *clarify the status of a known disease* (e.g. varices, Barrett's esophagus, inflammatory bowel disease);

Cotton and Williams' Practical Gastrointestinal Endoscopy: The Fundamentals, Eighth Edition.
Catharine M. Walsh, Ahmir Ahmad, Brian P. Saunders, Jonathan Cohen, Peter B. Cotton, and Christopher B. Williams.
© 2024 John Wiley & Sons Ltd. Published 2024 by John Wiley & Sons Ltd.
Companion website: www.wiley.com/go/cottonwilliams8e

3 *take specimens* (e.g. duodenal biopsy for malabsorption);

4 *screen for malignancy* and premalignancy in patients judged to be at increased risk of neoplasia (e.g. familial adenomatous polyposis);

5 *perform therapy* (e.g. hemostasis, dilatation, polypectomy, foreign body removal, tube placement).

Several of these indications may be combined: for example, diagnosis and therapy for acute bleeding, or classification and therapy for retreatment of known varices.

Guidelines about the appropriate use of endoscopy are published by endoscopy organizations. The "strength" of the indication in each circumstance will depend upon likely benefits from performing the proposed procedure, the perceived risks of the procedure and of forgoing the procedure, and any alternative approaches.

What are the potential adverse events?

The vast majority of endoscopic procedures go according to plan, but there are exceptions. Disappointments can include technical failures (inability to reach the desired area) and clinical failures (no benefit from the treatment). Here we focus on adverse events, previously called complications.

It is important to have agreed-upon definitions of adverse events, including when they are sufficiently notable to "count," and some assessment of their severity. An American Society for Gastrointestinal Endoscopy (ASGE) working group defined an adverse event as one that:

• prevents completion of the planned procedure (not simply a technical failure or poor preparation or toleration); and/or

• results in admission to hospital, prolongation of an existing hospital stay, another procedure (requiring sedation/anesthesia), or subsequent medical consultation.

Adverse events can be differentiated into pre-procedure, intra-procedure, post-procedure (up to 14 days), and late (after 14 days).

Unwanted events that do not rise to those levels are called "incidents." Examples include bleeding that is stopped by immediate endoscopic intervention, or transient hypoxia. These should be recorded for quality improvement, and also because some incidents (e.g. treated bleeding) increase the risk of subsequent events (e.g. re-bleeding).

Levels of severity for adverse events

Adverse events range from relatively minor to life-threatening, so it is necessary to have some measure of severity. Criteria for stratifying adverse events are outlined in Table 4.1.

Table 4.1 Severity grading system for adverse events (ASGE, 2010)

Mild
    Procedure aborted (or not started) because of an adverse event
    Post-procedure consult required by a different specialist
    Unplanned hospital admission required for less than 3 nights

Moderate
    Unplanned anesthesia/ventilation support
    Unplanned hospital admission for 4–10 nights
    ICU admission for 1 night
    Transfusion
    Repeat endoscopy to manage an adverse event
    Interventional endoscopy to manage an adverse event
    Interventional treatment for integument injuries

Severe
    Unplanned hospital admission for more than 10 nights
    ICU admission for more than one night
    Surgery to manage an adverse event
    Permanent disability (specify)

Fatal
    Death due to an adverse event

Rates of adverse events

Variable prior definitions and data collection methods, and a lack of community-based studies, make it difficult to quote precise statistics about the risks of endoscopy which will vary with the patient population as well as other factors. Although some of the most severe events (e.g. perforation, bleeding) are obvious immediately, others (e.g. transmission of infection) are delayed and difficult to track. However, large surveys suggest that the chance of suffering a severe adverse event after routine upper endoscopy is less than 1 in 1,000 cases. The risks are higher in the elderly and the acutely ill, and during therapeutic and emergency procedures. Inexperience, oversedation, and overconfidence are important contributory factors.

Specific adverse events

• *Hypoxia* should be detected early by careful nursing surveillance, aided by pulse oximetry, and treated quickly. Capnography can detect hypoventilation prior to the development of hypoxia.

• *Pulmonary aspiration* is probably more common than recognized. The risk is greater in patients with retained food residue (e.g. achalasia, pyloric stenosis), ascites, and in those with active bleeding.

• *Bleeding* may occur during and after endoscopy, from existing lesions (e.g. varices) or as a result of endoscopic manipulation (e.g. biopsy, polypectomy), or, occasionally, because of retching from a Mallory-Weiss tear. The risk of bleeding is greater in patients with coagulopathy, and in those taking anticoagulants and (possibly) antiplatelet agents.

• **Perforation** is the most feared adverse event of upper endoscopy but is rare. Perforation in the neck can occur in elderly patients, especially in the presence of a Zenker's diverticulum. The risk is minimized by gentle endoscope insertion under direct vision. Perforation beyond the cricopharyngeus is rare but can occur in patients who are undergoing therapeutic techniques such as stricture dilatation, polypectomy, or mucosal resection.

• **Cardiac dysrhythmias** are extremely rare. They require prompt recognition and expert treatment.

• **Infection.** Patients with active infections can pose risks to staff and to subsequent patients. Endoscopes (and accessories) are potential vehicles for the transmission of infection from patient to patient (e.g. *Helicobacter pylori,* salmonella, hepatitis, mycobacteria). This risk should be eliminated by assiduous attention to detail in cleaning and disinfection, and strict adherence to published guidelines and the manufacturer specifications, as outlined in Chapter 3. Endoscopy can provoke bacteremia, especially during therapeutic procedures such as dilatation. This may be dangerous in patients who are immunocompromised, and in some with diseased heart valves and prostheses. Antibiotic prophylaxis is advised in certain circumstances (see "Assessing and reducing specific risks" below).

Assessing and reducing specific risks

Certain comorbidities and medications clearly increase the risk of endoscopic procedures. A *checklist* should be used to ensure that all of the issues have been addressed. Some of this information must be obtained when the procedure is scheduled, as action is required days ahead of the procedure (e.g. adjusting anticoagulants). Other aspects are dealt with when the patient arrives in the pre-procedure area. Often decisions taken to minimize these risks require communication at the time of scheduling with the patient's other medical providers (e.g. cardiologist or internist) to develop an optimal plan based on a patient's medical conditions, and the anticipated specific risks of the endoscopic interventions planned.

• **Cardiac and pulmonary disease.** Patients with recent myocardial infarction, unstable angina, or hemodynamic instability are obviously at risk from any intervention. Expert advice should be sought from cardiologists. Endoscopy can be performed in patients with pacemakers and implantable cardioverter-defibrillators (ICDs), but the latter must be deactivated if diathermy is performed. Anesthetic supervision is essential if endoscopy is needed in such patients, and in others with respiratory insufficiency.

• **Coagulation disorders.** Patients with a known bleeding diathesis or coagulation disorder should have the situation normalized as far as possible before endoscopy (particularly if biopsy or polypectomy is likely). For patients on prescribed anticoagulation, the decision about whether to withhold or continue medications depends both on the bleeding risk of the intended endoscopic intervention and the patient-specific risks of stopping the anticoagulation. In those cases that require anticoagulants to be stopped ahead of time (e.g. polypectomy), patients at high risk for clotting while off medication can have their usual anticoagulation regime replaced by shorter-acting heparin for the period from before the procedure to early recovery, acting as a bridge until the resumed anticoagulation agent has taken effect. Others who are at lower risk for clotting while withholding anticoagulation can safely be managed without a heparin bridge. While certain oral antiplatelet drugs may need to be stopped in advance of endoscopy, there is little evidence that aspirin and nonsteroidal anti-inflammatory drugs increase the risk of adverse events. Those patients with cardiovascular disease on low-dose aspirin are generally advised not to stop this medication for endoscopy.

• *Sedation issues.* Anxious patients and others who have had prior problems with sedation can pose challenges for safe endoscopy. Individuals who are at risk of airway obstruction (e.g. known sleep apnea, obesity) or aspiration should undergo pre-endoscopy airway assessment. If in doubt, consider anesthesia support. Unsedated endoscopy is also a well-tolerated option in many patients and may be an option to consider.

• *Pregnancy.* Endoscopy is generally safe to perform during pregnancy. Nonetheless, it should only be done when there is a strong indication and after consultation with an obstetrician. When possible, postponement to the second trimester is best.

• *Infection.* The risk of developing endocarditis after upper and lower endoscopic procedures is extremely low, and there is no evidence that antibiotic prophylaxis is beneficial in that context. Antibiotic prophylaxis is generally recommended for patients undergoing percutaneous endoscopic gastrostomy (PEG) insertion, gastroscopy for upper GI bleeding in a cirrhotic patient, and for those with bacterial cholangitis having an ERCP. The American Heart Association delineated cardiac conditions associated with the highest risk of post-procedure infection, including:

- • prosthetic (mechanical or bioprosthetic) cardiac valves
- • history of previous endocarditis
- • cardiac transplant recipients who develop cardiac valvulopathy
- • patients with congenital heart disease (CHD)
- • those with unrepaired cyanotic CHD, including palliative shunts and conduits
- • those with completely repaired CHD with prosthetic material or devices, placed surgically or by catheter for the first 6 months after the procedure
- • those with repaired CHD with residual defects at the site or adjacent to the site of a prosthetic patch or device.

The local antibiotic policy should be documented in the endoscopy unit policy manual.

The American Society of Anesthesiologists (ASA) score is used in many units to describe broad categories of fitness for procedures and sedation (Table 4.2). Many recommend anesthesia assistance for patients with ASA scores of 3 or greater.

Table 4.2 ASA classification—anesthesia risk classes

Classification	Description	Adult examples	Pediatric examples
Class I	Healthy patient	Healthy (no acute or chronic disease), non-smoking	Healthy (no acute or chronic disease), normal BMI for age
Class II	Mild systemic disease without substantive functional limitations	Well-controlled hypertension, well-controlled diabetes mellitus, mild lung disease, smoker	Non-insulin-dependent diabetes mellitus, mild or moderate sleep apnea, asthma without exacerbations
Class III	Severe systemic disease with definite functional limitation	Poorly controlled diabetes mellitus, poorly controlled hypertension, history (>3 months) of myocardial infarction, morbid obesity	Poorly controlled epilepsy, insulin-dependent diabetes mellitus, morbid obesity, renal failure
Class IV	Severe systemic disease with acute, unstable symptoms	Recent (<3 months) myocardial infarction, acute renal failure or end-stage renal disease not undergoing regularly scheduled dialysis, severe respiratory distress, shock, sepsis	Symptomatic congenital cardiac abnormality, congestive heart failure, ventilator dependence, severe trauma
Class V	Severe systemic disease with imminent risk of death	Massive trauma, respiratory failure or arrest, decompensated congestive heart failure	Massive trauma, malignant hypertension, hepatic encephalopathy

Patient education and consent

Patients are entitled to be fully informed of the reasons why a procedure is recommended, the procedure's expected benefits and the potential risks, as well as the potential harms of forgoing the procedure, any limitations of the proposed procedure, and any alternatives. They also need to know exactly what will happen during the procedure, including any diagnostic or therapeutic interventions that may reasonably be anticipated to occur, and have the chance to ask questions. A discussion regarding the potential need for intubation, hospitalization and blood transfusion is important and the patient's preference should be documented. Additionally, off-label techniques and devices should be discussed as part of the informed consent process.

The ASGE recently recommended that informed consent may be obtained by any member of the GI team (including nurse, advanced practice provider, or trainee) who is thoroughly knowledgeable of and able to communicate the indication(s), risks, benefits, and alternatives of that procedure. It is clearly the specific endoscopist's responsibility to ensure that the process is concluded appropriately.

Ancillary materials

Information leaflets can facilitate the education process and should be given (or sent) to patients well in advance of the procedure, so that they can be studied carefully and digested. Suitable leaflets are available from national organizations, and on websites from expert centers. Examples are shown in Figs 4.1 and 4.2. They can be adapted or developed for local conditions. Some centers use videotapes and web-based instructional materials.

Upper endoscopy

Upper endoscopy is a common test, sometimes also called "Gastroscopy" or "EGD" (esophago-gastro-duodenoscopy). The endoscopist uses a medical instrument called an endoscope. It is a long, thin, flexible tube with a light and tiny camera at the end.

The endoscopist passes the endoscope through your mouth to examine the lining of the upper digestive system—the esophagus, stomach, and duodenum. The camera transmits live pictures of your insides to a television screen for the endoscopist and team to examine and record.

Endoscopy is the best way to find (and to rule out) inflammation, narrowings, ulcers, and tumors. Endoscopists can treat many of these conditions at the same time through the endoscope.

How do I prepare?

Do not eat anything for 6 hours before the test. You may drink clear fluids until 2 hours before the test and take blood pressure and heart medicines in the morning, with a sip of water. Tell your endoscopist/endoscopy team if you:
• Have any allergies, heart or breathing problems.
• Are taking insulin for diabetes.
• Have had an endoscopy in the past and had any problems.
• Are or might be pregnant.
• Take medicines that thin the blood (anticoagulants). These may need to be stopped or changed.
• Use a CPAP machine.
• Have a pacemaker or internal defibrillator.

Bring any records of past endoscopy tests if you have them.

Make sure an adult can accompany you and take you home. The sedating medicines that you will be given do not wear out completely for several hours. You will NOT be able to drive.

What will happen?

Your endoscopist and endoscopy team members will talk to you about the test and answer any questions you may have. You should know why the test is being recommended, its expected benefits, potential risks, limitations, and any alternatives. You will be asked to sign a consent form that shows that you understand and wish to go ahead.

You will be asked to put on a gown and remove eyeglasses, contact lenses, and any dentures. The nurse will set up an intravenous (IV) line in your arm, and put a blood pressure cuff on your arm and an oxygen monitor clip on a finger.

Fig 4.1 Sample patient information leaflet for upper endoscopy.

Most patients are given medicines through the IV to make you very sleepy and less aware of the test. A numbing throat spray is sometimes used. Occasionally, full anesthesia is needed. You will be taken on a stretcher into the endoscopy room.

The endoscopist will place a plastic guard between your teeth and pass the endoscope though it into your mouth. When you swallow it will pass easily into your esophagus, like food. The endoscope will not interfere with your breathing. The endoscopist will then advance the endoscope to examine the stomach and duodenum. He/she may take specimens (biopsies) for laboratory analysis and perform any necessary treatments. The endoscope is then removed. The test takes 10–20 minutes, longer if treatments are done.

Afterwards

You will wake up quickly in the recovery area. The nurse will remove the IV and let you get dressed and take a drink of water. The endoscopist will tell you what he/she found and did. It is important that someone is with you during this conversation, as the medicines dull your immediate memory. The staff will give you written instructions to follow at home and any further appointments.

You MUST NOT drive home and should not make any important decisions or use machinery until the next day. You may resume normal diet and medications but should avoid alcohol and sleeping pills.

Your throat may be a little sore and the air that the endoscopist puts into your stomach to see better may make you feel bloated.

Risks?

Upper endoscopy is a very safe procedure, but, as the team has explained to you beforehand, there are risks. These vary according to your own health status and particular clinical problem, and whether treatment is done during the procedure. Something sufficient to keep you in hospital for treatment may occur in about 1:500 cases, such as heart or chest problems, bleeding, and tearing of the wall (perforation). Surgery may be needed.

Call your care team if you:
- Have severe pain
- Are vomiting
- Pass or vomit blood
- Have chills or fever above 101°F (38°C).

In emergency, call the GI doctor on call at . . .
This information is provided as an educational service, and is not a substitute for professional medical care.

Fig 4.1 Continued.

Colonoscopy

Colonoscopy is a common test. The endoscopist uses a medical instrument called an endoscope. It is a long, thin, flexible tube with a light and tiny camera at the end.

The endoscopist passes the endoscope through your anus to examine the lining of the rectum and colon. The camera transmits live pictures of your insides to a television screen for the endoscopist and team to examine and record.

Colonoscopy is the best way to find (and to rule out) inflammation, narrowings, and tumors/polyps. Endoscopist can treat many of these conditions at the same time through the endoscope.

How do I prepare?

Your colon needs to be completely clean for the exam. You will receive detailed instructions about the necessary preparation. Do not eat from midday the day before your procedure (unless advised otherwise) and continue to drink clear fluids until 2 hours before the test. You may take blood pressure and heart medicines in the morning, with a sip of water.

Tell your endoscopist/endoscopy team if you:
• Have any allergies or heart or breathing problems.
• Are taking insulin for diabetes.
• Have had an endoscopy in the past and had any problems.
• Are or might be pregnant.
• Take medicines that thin the blood (anticoagulants). These may need to be stopped or changed.
• Use a CPAP machine.
• Have a pacemaker or internal defibrillator.

Bring any records of past endoscopy tests if you have them.

Make sure an adult can accompany you and take you home. The sedating medicines that you will be given do not wear out completely for several hours. You will NOT be able to drive.

What will happen?

Your endoscopist and endoscopy team members will talk to you about the test and answer any questions. You should know why the test is being recommended, its expected benefits, potential risks, limitations, and any alternatives. You will be asked to sign a consent form that shows that you understand and wish to go ahead.

You will be asked to put on a gown and remove eyeglasses, contact lenses, and any dentures. The nurse will set up an intravenous (IV) line in your arm, and put a blood pressure cuff on your arm and an oxygen monitor clip on a finger.

Fig 4.2 Sample patient information leaflet for colonoscopy.

Although some patients have colonoscopy without any sedation, most opt to have medicines through the IV to make them very sleepy and less aware of the test. Occasionally, full anesthesia is needed. Your endoscopist will advise. You will be taken on a stretcher into the endoscopy room.

When you are sleepy, the endoscopist will do a rectal exam. He/she will then pass the endoscope though your anus, into the rectum and gradually around the colon. You may feel some cramping during the procedure. The endoscopist may take specimens (biopsies) for laboratory analysis and will perform any necessary treatments. The endoscope is then removed. The test takes 15–30 minutes, sometimes longer if treatments are done.

Afterwards

You will wake up quickly in the recovery area. The nurse will remove the IV and let you get dressed and take a drink of water. The endoscopist will tell you what he/she found and did. It is important that someone is with you during this conversation, as the medicines dull your immediate memory. The staff will give you a report of the exam, written instructions to follow at home, and any further appointments.

You MUST NOT drive home and should not make any important decisions or use machinery until the next day. You may resume normal diet and medications but should avoid alcohol and sleeping pills.
The air that the endoscopist puts into your colon to see better may make you feel bloated.

Risks?

Colonoscopy is a safe procedure, but, as the team has explained to you beforehand, there are risks. These vary according to your own health status and particular clinical problem, and what is done during the procedure. Bleeding can occur for up to two weeks after some treatments, like removing a polyp. It may need a second colonoscopy to stop it. Something sufficient to keep you in hospital for treatment may occur in about 1:500 cases, such as heart or chest problems, and tearing of the colon wall (perforation). Surgery may be needed.

Call your care team if you:

• Have severe pain
• Are vomiting
• Pass blood
• Have chills or fever above 101°F (38°C).

In emergency, call the GI doctor on call at . . .

This information is provided as an educational service and is not a substitute for professional medical advice.

Fig 4.2 Continued.

Consent form

Patients must be given the opportunity to ask questions before being invited to confirm their understanding and agreement to the procedure by signing the consent form in the presence of a witness. This document simply confirms that the patient truly understands and accepts what is being proposed, including the potential for harm. For pediatric patients, developmentally appropriate consent and assent (a child's affirmative agreement) processes should be used that incorporate age-appropriate language and materials.

The very simplicity and safety of upper endoscopy may tempt busy endoscopy teams to hurry the consent process. That is not good medical practice and carries medicolegal risk.

Physical preparation

Before upper endoscopy the patient should prepare by not eating for 6 hours (usually overnight) ahead of the procedure, with clear fluids allowed up to 2 hours beforehand. A series of medical checks and actions to optimize the safety of the intervention are undertaken, including a general medical review, confirmation of current medication, assessment of vital signs and cardiopulmonary status, and attention to the many details concerning risks and risk reduction as detailed above. Intravenous (IV) access should be established, preferably in the right arm or hand. Spectacles, dentures, and jewelry (including in body piercings) should be removed and stored safely. Consultation with a nurse is helpful with regard to adjustment of chronic medications (e.g. insulin and antihypertensives) the night before or on the morning of the procedure.

Sedation/anesthesia

Sedation practice varies widely around the world. Routine (diagnostic) upper endoscopy can be performed without any sedation, using only pharyngeal anesthesia. Although the avoidance of sedation has obvious advantages in terms of safety and fast recovery, most patients in industrialized countries expect and receive some degree of sedation/analgesia. Some require full anesthesia.

Monitoring

Sedation and other medications are given by the endoscopist or by the endoscopy nurse under supervision. The nurse is the practical guardian of the patient's safety and comfort during endoscopic procedures. Nursing surveillance should be supplemented with monitoring devices, at least for heart rate, blood pressure, and oxygen saturation. Supplemental oxygen is used routinely in many units, although some argue that this may mask hypoventilation, which is better detected by monitoring of carbon dioxide (capnography). Ventilatory activity and the level of consciousness and discomfort should also be visually assessed. Electrocardiographic monitoring is generally recommended for prolonged procedures and patients at high risk, including the elderly and patients with significant cardiovascular or pulmonary disease or a history of dysrhythmias.

The nurse should document this process carefully, along with the patient's vital signs, monitoring data, and the patient's response. Emergency drugs and equipment must be available nearby, and the endoscopist should be trained in resuscitation and life support.

Levels of sedation

Moderate sedation (formally referred to as ***conscious sedation***) is intended to make unpleasant procedures tolerable for patients, while maintaining their ability to self-ventilate, maintain a clear airway, and respond to light physical stimulation and verbal commands. Endoscopists giving moderate sedation must be fully familiar with the techniques and dosing. Many centers mandate specific training, and credentialing, for moderate sedation. The training is given by anesthesiologists. In contrast to conscious sedation, in ***deep sedation*** the patient cannot be easily aroused, and there may be partial or complete loss of protective reflexes, including the ability to maintain a patent airway. This level of sedation requires anesthesia supervision. However, in contrast with general anesthesia, a patient under deep sedation can respond purposefully to painful stimuli.

Sedation/analgesic agents (Table 4.3)
Anxiolytics

Short-acting benzodiazepines are commonly administered by slow IV injection/titration. Midazolam (Versed®), with its fast onset of action, short duration of action, and high amnestic properties, makes an ideal choice. It is given in an initial dose of 0.5–2 mg, with increments of 0.5–1 mg every 2–10 minutes, to a maximum of about 5 mg. Doses are determined by the patient's age, weight, medical and drug history, and by their response.

Table 4.3 Commonly used sedation/analgesic agents.

Sedation/analgesic agents*	Initial IV dose	Onset	Duration of effect
Midazolam	0.5–2 mg	1–5 min	1–2 h
Diazepam	1–5 mg	1–5 min	2–6 h
Meperidine (pethidine)	25–50 mg	2–5 min	2–4 h
Fentanyl	50–100 µg	1 min	20–60 min
Diphenhydramine	10–50 mg	1–10 min	2–6 h
Droperidol	1–5 mg	5–10 min	2–4 h
Reversal agents			
Flumazenil (for benzodiazepines)	0.1–0.2 mg	30–60 s	30–60 min
Naloxone (for opioids)	0.2–0.4 mg (IV and IM)	1–2 min	45 min

* For sedation purposes 25–50% increments of the initial dose can be administered every 2–10 minutes. Dosages should be adjusted according to patient age, body weight, medical history, and concomitant drug use.

Narcotics

Narcotic analgesics are often given with benzodiazepines, but the combination increases the risk of respiratory depression. Meperidine (pethidine) is given in an initial dose of 25–50 mg, with increments of 25 mg up to a maximum of 100 mg, but can cause venous irritation and is relatively long-lasting. Its use has mainly been replaced by more modern short-acting opiates such as fentanyl (Sublimaze®), which has a rapid onset of action and clearance and reduced incidence of venous irritation and nausea compared with meperidine. Fentanyl is usually given in an initial dose of 50 μg, with increments of 25 μg up to a maximum of 100 μg.

Antagonists

Opioids can be reversed by naloxone, given both intramuscularly (IM) and IV. Benzodiazepines are reversed by flumazenil, given by slow IV injection. Both antagonists have shorter half-lives than the drugs they antagonize.

Other medications

Pharyngeal anesthesia (given by spray) is used in many units to suppress the gag reflex during endoscopy. The patient should not be asked to say "ah" when applying the spray because this exposes the larynx to the anesthesia, which may suppress the cough reflex. Some endoscopists avoid local anesthesia when using sedation, believing that it may increase the risk of aspiration. Topical benzocaine spray is avoided due to its association with methemoglobinemia.

Excessive intestinal contraction can be suppressed with IV injections of *glucagon* (increments of 0.25 mg up to 2 mg) or *hyoscine butylbromide* (Buscopan®) 20–40 mg in countries where it is available.

Silicone-containing emulsions—either swallowed beforehand or injected down the channel—can be used to suppress foaming.

Anesthesia

There are circumstances in which the presence of an anesthesiologist is helpful, and sometimes full anesthesia is required. Examples include patients who are difficult to sedate, heavy drinkers, those with high ASA scores, concerns about airway protection or risk of aspiration, or the expected duration and complexity of the procedure planned. Anesthesiologist-directed sedation should be used for children.

Propofol (Diprivan®) is a useful short-acting anesthesia agent that seems ideal for endoscopic procedures. It has a mild amnestic effect and no analgesic effect and therefore is often used in conjunction with a short-acting opiate and benzodiazepine. In most centers and countries this can be given only by anesthesiologists.

Numerous other sedation/anesthesia practices have been tested and used, such as patient-controlled nitrous oxide and acupuncture.

Pregnancy and lactation

While this area has not been extensively studied, meperidine (pethidine) alone is preferred for procedural sedation during pregnancy. Although there is evidence of risk to the fetus with Midazolam (category D, Food and Drug Administration), it can be used in small doses in combination with meperidine as needed. If deep sedation is required, it should be performed by an anesthesiologist.

Concentrations of sedatives and analgesics vary in breast milk after procedural administration. In general, breast-feeding may be continued after fentanyl administration, which is preferred over meperidine during lactation. Infants should not be breast-fed for at least 4 hours following maternal administration of midazolam.

Recovery and discharge

After the endoscope is removed, the assisting nurse checks on the status of the patient and then transfers care to the recovery area staff. Monitoring is continued until the patient is fully awake, usually 20–30 minutes after standard sedation. A longer period of observation may be necessary after deep sedation or full general anesthesia. Significant patient complaints in the recovery area must be conveyed to the endoscopist with documentation of any evaluation or planned response to ensure that an adverse event has not occurred.

The patient will appreciate a drink after sedation once any pharyngeal anesthesia has worn off. When established discharge criteria have been met, the patient gets dressed and the endoscopic findings and follow-up plan are discussed. Endoscopy is not complete until the patient has been counseled about the findings, their implications, and resulting plans, as well as plans for conveying the pathology results. This is a key opportunity for communication with the patient to ensure that proper follow-up ensues; inclusion of a written list of findings in the discharge materials or a copy of the completed procedure note may facilitate this process. If sedation has been given, it is essential that this process takes place in the presence of an accompanying person, because of the potential for significant delayed amnesia. In addition, the patient should be instructed to have a responsible person to escort them home. They should not be allowed to drive, make important medicolegal decisions, or operate heavy machinery.

Discharge instructions should be given in writing, including details of:
- resumption of diet and activities;
- medications to be restarted, stopped, and commenced;
- further appointments;
- how pathology results will be communicated;
- symptoms to report (and who to contact), including severe pain, distension, fever, vomiting, or passing blood.

Some units also print out and provide patient education materials relevant to the specific endoscopic findings.

Managing adverse events

Careful attention to all of these safeguards and cautions will help to ensure that most procedures proceed smoothly. Nevertheless, unplanned events do occur, even in the best of hands and environments, and it is natural for endoscopists and staff to feel bad when things "go wrong," especially when they are severe or life-threatening.

The most important action is to prepare for, recognize, and manage these situations appropriately. The well-informed patient (and relatives) will have been told and should know that bad things can happen. This is an integral and important part of the communication and consent process, so it is appropriate and correct to address adverse events in that spirit. For example: "It looks like we have a perforation here. Remember that this was mentioned as a remote possibility beforehand, and I'm sorry that it has occurred. This is what we need to do."

Saying "sorry it happened" (not "sorry I messed up somehow") shows that you care, and is very important to support the provider-patient relationship. It is helpful to have a colleague present for this conversation.

Your distress is understandable and worthy, and you need to be sympathetic, but it is important to also be professional and matter of fact. Never attempt to cover up the facts. Document what has happened and communicate widely—with the patient, interested relatives, referring doctors, supervisors, and your risk management office.

Act quickly. Delay in managing adverse events is foolish and can be dangerous, both medically and legally. Get appropriate radiographs and lab studies, expert advice, and a surgical opinion (from a surgeon who understands the issues) for anything that might require surgical intervention. Sometimes it may be wise to offer transfer of the patient to a colleague or to a larger center, but if this happens try to keep in touch and to show continuing interest and concern. Patients (and relatives) do not like to feel abandoned.

The best protection against medicolegal jeopardy is to communicate carefully and, above all, to show that you care.

Further reading

Guidelines on indications, sedation, risks, and risk reduction can be found at www.asge.org/home/resources/key-resources/guidelines, https://www.bsg.org.uk/resource-type/clinical-resources/guidelines/, and many other sources.

Adverse events

Cotton PB, Eisen G, Aabakken L, et al. A lexicon for endoscopic adverse events: Report of an ASGE workshop. *Gastrointest Endosc* 2010;71(3): 446–54.

Cotton PB, Eisen G, Romagnuolo J, et al. Grading the complexity of endoscopic procedures: Results of an ASGE working party. *Gastrointest Endosc* 2011;73(5):868–74.

Romagnuolo J, Cotton PB, Eisen G, et al. Identifying and reporting risk factors for adverse events in endoscopy. Part I: Cardiopulmonary events. *Gastrointest Endosc* 2011;73(3):579–85.

Romagnuolo J, Cotton PB, Eisen G, et al. Identifying and reporting risk factors for adverse events in endoscopy. Part II: Noncardiopulmonary events. *Gastrointest Endosc* 2011;73(3):586–97.

Antibiotic prophylaxis

ASGE Standards of Practice Committee, Khashab MA, Chithandi KV, et al. Antibiotic prophylaxis for GI endoscopy. *Gastrointest Endosc* 2015;81(1):81–9.

Allison MC, Sandoe JAT, Tighe R, et al. Antibiotic prophylaxis in gastrointestinal endoscopy. *Gut* 2009;58(6):869–80.

Quality

Beg S, Ragunath K, Wyman A, et al. Quality standards in upper gastrointestinal endoscopy: A position statement of the British Society of Gastroenterology (BSG) and Association of Upper Gastrointestinal Surgeons of Great Britain and Ireland (AUGIS). *Gut* 2017;66(11): 1886–99.

Bisschops R, Areia A, Coron E, et al. Performance measures for upper gastrointestinal endoscopy: A European Society of Gastrointestinal Endoscopy quality improvement initiative. *Endoscopy* 2016;48(9): 843–64.

Park WG, Shaheen NJ, Cohen J, et al. Quality indicators for EGD. *Gastrointest Endosc* 2015;81(1):17–30.

Consent

Storm AC, Fishman DS, Buxbaum JL, et al. American Society for Gastrointestinal Endoscopy guideline on informed consent for GI endoscopic procedures. *Gastrointest Endosc* 2022;95(2):207–15.

Everett SM, Griffiths H, Nandosoma U, et al. Guideline for obtaining valid consent for gastrointestinal endoscopy procedures. *Gut* 2016;65(10): 1585–601.

Anticoagulation

Veitch AM, Radaelli F, Alikhan R. et al. Endoscopy in patients on antiplatelet or anticoagulant therapy: British Society of Gastroenterology (BSG) and European Society of Gastrointestinal Endoscopy (ESGE) guideline update. *Gut* 2021;70(9):1611–28.

Sedation

ASGE Standards of Practice Committee, Early DS, Lightdale JR, et al. Guidelines for sedation and anesthesia in GI endoscopy. *Gastrointest Endosc* 2018;87(2):327–37.

American Association for the Study of Liver Diseases, American College of Gastroenterology, American Gastroenterological Association Institute, et al. Multisociety sedation curriculum for gastrointestinal endoscopy. *Gastrointest Endosc* 2012;76(1):e1–e25.

Turnbull D, Gannon J, Krovvidi H. Guidelines for the provision of anaesthesia services in the non-theatre environment (chapter 7). In: *Guidelines for the Provision of Anaesthesia Services*. London, United Kingdom: Royal College of Anaesthetists, 2021. Available at: https://www.rcoa.ac.uk/gpas/chapter-7.

CHAPTER 5

Upper Endoscopy: The Fundamentals

Details of patient preparation are given in Chapter 4, along with some discussion of indications and risks. Both the endoscopist and the patient must be confident that the procedure is likely to be worthwhile and that it will be performed skillfully, with appropriate equipment and assistance.

Patient position

The patient lies on the examination trolley/stretcher in the left lateral decubitus position with the intravenous access line preferably in the *right* arm. The patient's head is supported on a small, firm pillow or doughnut-shaped headrest, so as to remain in a comfortable neutral position (Fig 5.1).

Monitoring devices are attached, and supplemental oxygen is given, usually via nasal prongs. Necessary sedation and/or pharyngeal anesthesia is applied. A biteguard is placed.

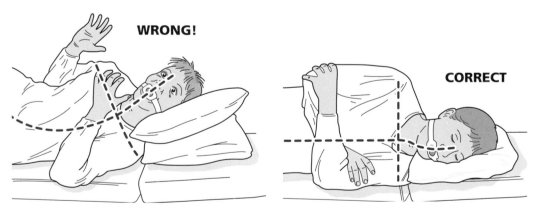

Fig 5.1 Preparing the patient correctly for upper gastrointestinal endoscopy.

Cotton and Williams' Practical Gastrointestinal Endoscopy: The Fundamentals, Eighth Edition.
Catharine M. Walsh, Ahmir Ahmad, Brian P. Saunders, Jonathan Cohen, Peter B. Cotton, and Christopher B. Williams.
© 2024 John Wiley & Sons Ltd. Published 2024 by John Wiley & Sons Ltd.
Companion website: www.wiley.com/go/cottonwilliams8e

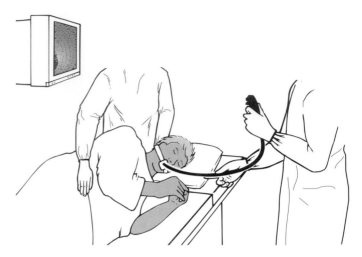

Fig 5.2 A neutral body posture and balanced stance with a straight instrument, gently handled.

Middle "helper" finger

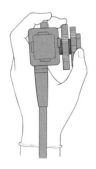

Fig 5.3 The thumb rests on the up/down angulation control knob with the first finger on the air/water valve; the middle finger can also assist with knob steering. The umbilicus is draped on the inside of the forearm to facilitate the application of torque.

Fig 5.4 The thumb can reach across to the left/right angulation control knob.

Endoscopist position

A neutral body posture is essential to minimize strain on the endoscopist's upper body during endoscopy and the risk of injury over time. The video monitor should be adjusted such that it is directly in front of the endoscopist, at a distance of 52–182 cm, with the center of the monitor at resting eye position, 15–25 degrees below the horizon, to prevent neck strain. The height of the bed should be adjusted for the endoscopist's comfort, positioned between elbow height and 10 cm below elbow height to allow for a working range of the forearms between 0 and 10 degrees below the elbows. For upper endoscopy, the endoscopic processer should ideally be behind the endoscopist such that the patient's mouth is at the level of (and in line with) the insertion of the endoscope into the processer.

Endoscope handling

The endoscopist should stand comfortably facing the patient, holding the instrument so that it runs in a gentle curve to the patient's mouth (Fig 5.2).

The control head of the endoscope should be placed in the palm of the left hand and held between the fourth and fifth fingers and the base of the thumb, with the tip of the thumb resting on the up/down angulation control knob and the umbilicus inside of the forearm to facilitate the application of torque (i.e. rotation along the longitudinal axis) (Fig 5.3). This grip leaves the first finger free to activate the air/water and suction buttons. The second (middle) finger assists the thumb as a helper or "ratchet" during major movements of the up/down control. Some people can also manage the left/right angulation control knob with the left thumb (Fig 5.4). During upper endoscopy, the endoscopist can apply torque along the longitudinal shaft of the endoscope by moving the left arm and hand and/or body: an important part of steering.

The right hand is used to push and pull the instrument, and to control accessories such as biopsy forceps.

Passing the endoscope

Select a standard forward-viewing endoscope and check it. Perform a white-light balance (where necessary), lubricate the distal tip, and double-check the critical functions:
- tip angulation
- CO_2/air and water
- suction
- image quality.

Check that the patient is stable and comfortable, and that the endoscopy assistant is ready. When sedated, patients may slump into positions in which swallowing anything is a challenge. The patient should be facing directly in front, with the neck slightly flexed. Most endoscopists pass instruments under direct vision. Sometimes it may be necessary to insert the endoscope blindly, or with finger guidance.

Direct vision insertion

Insertion under direct vision is the best and standard method.

1 *Hold the endoscope comfortably*—the head with the left hand, and the shaft with the right hand at the 25 cm mark; holding the endoscope head at waist level will help ensure that the shaft is in the horizontal plane to facilitate intubation.

2 *Rehearse up/down movement of the controls* to ensure that the angulated bending section will move in the correct longitudinal axis to follow the pharynx (Fig 5.5). Adjust the lateral angulation control or torque the shaft appropriately so that the scope will travel down the midline.

3 *Pass the tip of the endoscope through the biteguard and over the tongue*, initially looking at the patient, not at the monitor.

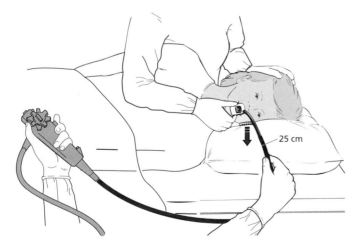

Fig 5.5 The endoscopist pre-rehearses tip angulation in the correct axis before insertion. Holding the endoscope head with the left hand at waist level will help ensure that the shaft is in the horizontal plane to facilitate intubation.

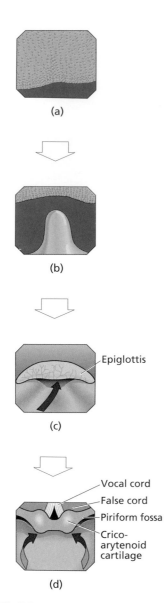

Fig 5.6 (a) Follow the center of the tongue . . . (b) . . . past the uvula . . . (c) . . . and the epiglottis . . . (d) . . . to pass below the cricoarytenoid into the piriform fossa, preferably on the left side.

4 Gently angulate the tip "up" (with your left thumb on the up/down angulation control knob) as it passes over the tongue.

5 *Now look at the monitor.* Look for a rough, pale surface of the tongue horizontally in the upper (anterior) part of the view and keep the interface between it and the red surface of the palate in the center of view by deflecting the endoscope tip up (toward 12 o'clock) as required, while advancing inward over the curve of the tongue.

6 *Stay in the midline* by watching for the linear "median raphe" of the tongue or the convexity of its midpart (Fig 5.6a), correcting if necessary, by rotating the shaft. The uvula is often seen transiently, projected *upward* in the lower part of the monitor view (Fig 5.6b).

7 *Advance gently.* The epiglottis and then the cricoarytenoid cartilage with the "false" vocal cords above it (and the vocal cords 2–3 cm beyond) are visible in the upper part of the view (Fig 5.6c).

8 *The first, or pharyngeal, part of the esophagus is in tonic contraction* and so is seen only transiently during swallowing. To reach it, angle the tip downward (posteriorly) so that the scope tip comes into a more neutral position and the tip passes inferior to the curve of the cricoarytenoid cartilage and into the piriform fossa. In keeping with gravity, when a patient is in the left lateral position, it is preferable to advance along the left side of the pyriform fossa. However, if several attempts to insert the scope have failed, advancement into the right-sided piriform fossa should be attempted; avoid the midline as the bulge of the cartilage against the cervical spine makes central passage difficult (Fig 5.6d), and push *gently* inward.

9 *There is often a "red-out"* as the tip impacts into the cricopharyngeal sphincter; insufflate air, maintain **gentle** inward pressure, ask the patient to swallow if they are alert, and the instrument should slip into the esophagus within a few seconds. If necessary, ask the patient to swallow again, pushing gently as the sphincter opens.

10 *Keep watching carefully* to ensure smooth mucosal "slide-by" as the instrument passes semi-blind into the upper esophagus, for this is where a diverticulum may occur.

11 Throughout this process:
- *be gentle*, feel the tube slide in
- *insufflation can be useful* to help open the upper esophagus
- *coordinate gentle onward pressure with the patient's attempts to swallow*
- *if alert, encourage the patient*, e.g. "swallow, swallow again, well done . . . now take deep breaths." This is best done by the endoscopist alone. Too many voices may confuse the patient and may suggest a degree of panic.

12 If the view is lost, or a bulging tongue deflects the scope, or the teeth are seen, withdraw the endoscope and start again.

13 *Be gentle*; force is dangerous and unnecessary (Video 5.1).

Blind insertion

This technique (originating from the time when most gastroscopes were side-viewing and were still used for endoscopic retrograde cholangiopancreatography [ERCP] insertions) is a slight variation of the better direct vision method but is done mainly by feel and by watching the patient, rather than by looking at the endoscopic view on the monitor. The assistant maintains the patient's neck slightly flexed. The endoscopist passes the instrument tip through the biteguard and over the tongue to the back of the mouth; using the left thumb on the up/down angulation control knob, the tip is then actively deflected "upward" so that it curls in the midline over the back of the tongue and into the midline of the pharynx. The tip is advanced slightly and angled down a little, and the thumb is then removed from the tip control. Slight forward pressure is maintained, and the patient is asked to swallow as the 20 cm mark approaches the biteguard. There is an obvious feeling of "give" as the tip passes the cricopharyngeal sphincter and then slides easily into the esophagus.

Insertion with tubes in place

Endotracheal tubes present no problem for the endoscopist inserting under direct vision, the scope being angled down posterior to the tube and gently pushed through the cricopharyngeal sphincter. Deflating the cuff of the tube may be occasionally necessary to allow easier passage, especially with larger instruments. An existing nasogastric tube may be a useful guide to the lumen. Withdrawing the endoscope may displace a nasogastric or nasoenteric tube, but this risk can be minimized by stiffening the tube with a guidewire.

Finger-assisted insertion

This method is inelegant, and is needed only rarely, when standard methods fail. The control head of the instrument is held by an assistant (avoiding contact with the angulation controls). The biteguard is fitted over the shaft before insertion. The endoscopist puts the second and third fingers of the left hand over the back of the tongue. With the right hand, the tip of the instrument is passed over the tongue, and the inserted fingers of the left hand are used to guide it into the midline of the pharynx (Fig 5.7). The fingers are

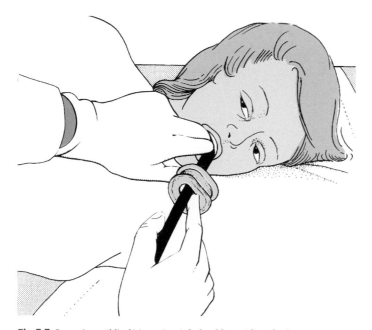

Fig 5.7 Sometimes "blind" insertion is helped by guiding the instrument between two fingers.

withdrawn, the biteguard is slid into place, and the patient is asked to swallow. If swallowing is not effective, the tip of the instrument has probably fallen into the left pyriform fossa.

Routine diagnostic survey

Whatever the precise indication, it is usually appropriate to examine the entire esophagus, stomach, and proximal duodenum, wherever possible. A complete survey may sometimes be prevented by stricturing from disease or previous surgery, or can be curtailed for other reasons.

It is important to develop a systematic routine to reduce the possibility of missing any area.

• *Always advance the instrument under direct vision*, using insufflation and suction as required, and slowing as necessary during active peristalsis.

• *Mucosal views are often optimal during instrument withdrawal*, when the organs are fully distended with air, but inspection during insertion is also important, as minor trauma by the instrument tip (or excessive suction) may produce small mucosal lesions with consequent diagnostic confusion.

• *Lesions noted during insertion are best examined in detail* (and sampled for histology or cytology) following a complete routine survey of other areas.

• *As well as being systematic in survey, be precise in movements and decisive in making a "mental map"* of what is being seen. A careful and complete examination can be achieved in less than 7–10 minutes by avoiding unnecessary movements and repeated examinations of the same area.

Golden rules for endoscopic safety:

• *do not push if you cannot see*
• *if in doubt, insufflate and pull back*.

Esophagus

Straighten out the tip of the endoscope as you advance the endoscope down the esophagus and apply slight tip deflection and insufflation as required to maintain a clear mucosal view. It is important to advance the endoscope slowly to allow for examination of the esophageal contour and mucosa.

The esophagus (Fig 5.8) extends:

• from the cricopharyngeal sphincter
• behind the left main bronchus, the left atrium, and aorta
• to the gastroesophageal (G-E) mucosal junction, which is usually easy to identify at 38–40 cm from the incisor teeth (in adults) as the point where pale pink squamous esophageal mucosa abuts darker red columnar gastric mucosa. This squamocolumnar junction is often irregular and therefore can also be called the "Z-line." The gastroesophageal junction should be situated at the top of the gastric folds in a semi-inflated esophagus. Pink mucosa extending cephalad from the top of the gastric folds suggests Barrett's esophagus; biopsies are required to establish the diagnosis and exclude dysplasia.

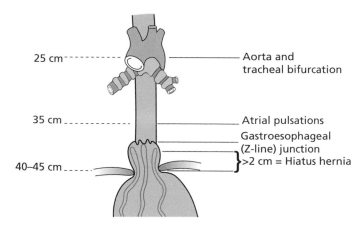

25 cm········· — Aorta and
tracheal bifurcation

35 cm··········· — Atrial pulsations

Gastroesophageal
(Z-line) junction
}>2 cm = Hiatus hernia

40–45 cm······

Fig 5.8 Esophageal landmarks—with a small hiatal hernia.

The diaphragmatic hiatus normally clasps the esophagus at or just below the gastroesophageal junction. The position of the hiatus can be highlighted by asking the patient to sniff or to take deep breaths and is recorded as the distance from the incisors. In any patient, the precise relationship of the Z-line to the diaphragmatic hiatus varies somewhat during an endoscopy (depending on the patient's position, respiration, and gastric distension). In normal patients, the gastric mucosa is often seen up to 1 cm above the diaphragm. A *hiatus hernia* is diagnosed if the Z-line remains more than 2 cm above the hiatus. From the clinical point of view, however, the presence or degree of herniation may be less important than any resulting esophageal lesions (e.g. esophagitis or the columnar transformation of Barrett's).

Hiatal hernias are most often axial or "sliding," in which the gastroesophageal junction, and sometimes the cardia, "slide" above the diaphragm. Other parts of the stomach may, less commonly, move above the diaphragm into the mediastinum alongside the esophagus in what is called a paraesophageal hiatus hernia (Fig 5.9).

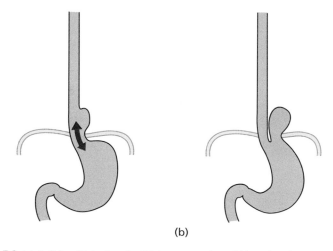

(a)   (b)

Fig 5.9 (a) A sliding hiatus hernia. (b) A paraoesophageal hiatus hernia.

Assessment of the diaphragmatic hiatus is facilitated by examining the way the flap valve pinches the scope when viewed from the endoscope tip when it is retroflexed in the stomach looking back up at the gastroesophageal junction. The favored method of grading hiatus hernias is by retroflexed views and the Hill classification (Fig 5.10). In Hill I there is a fold or flap valve with tight closure around the endoscope; in Hill II the fold is less marked, with respiration-dependent incomplete closure; Hill III shows no obvious fold and no closure; and in Hill IV there is permanent opening of the gastroesophageal junction.

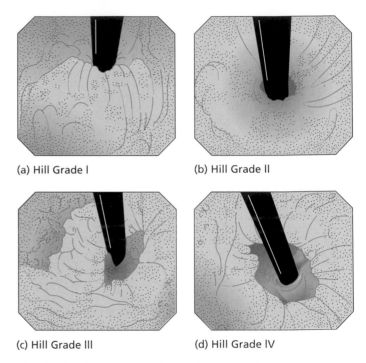

(a) Hill Grade I

(b) Hill Grade II

(c) Hill Grade III

(d) Hill Grade IV

Fig 5.10 The Hill classification whereby the gastroesophageal flap valve is inspected in retroflexion and classified into one of four grades

Stomach

In the absence of stenosis, the endoscope can be advanced easily through the cardia and into the stomach under direct vision. The distal esophagus usually angles to the patient's left posterior side as it passes through the diaphragm, so it may be necessary to rotate the instrument tip counterclockwise slightly to remain in the correct axis (Fig 5.11). Unless the cardia is unduly lax, the mucosal view is lost momentarily as the tip passes through, with the passage being felt by the advancing hand as a slight "give." If the tip is further advanced in the same plane, it will abut on the posterior wall of the upper body of the stomach, leading to red-out. Pushing in blindly also risks retroflexing toward the cardia. Thus:

1 *torque the endoscope counterclockwise ("left turn") by dropping the endoscopist's left hand slightly downward* to avoid hitting the upper body of the stomach (Fig 5.11), and insufflate as the endoscope tip passes through the cardia

2 *if there is no clear luminal view, withdraw slightly* to disimpact the tip from the wall of the fundus or from the pool of gastric juice on the greater curve

3 *the endoscopic view is predictable* with the patient in the left lateral position and the instrument head held upright (Figs 5.12 and 5.13); the smooth lesser curvature is on the endoscopist's right with the angulus distally, the longitudinal folds of the greater curve are to the left and its posterior aspect is below

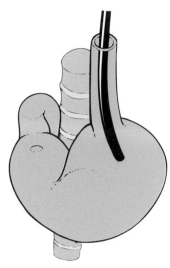

Fig 5.11 The distal esophagus angles the scope into the posterior wall of the upper body of the stomach. Application of counterclockwise torque will help to overcome this.

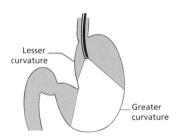

Fig 5.12 With the gastroscope high on the lesser curve . . .

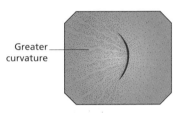

Fig 5.13 . . . the view is of the angulus in the distance, with the greater curve longitudinal folds. A fluid pool is often on the left.

4 *aspirate any pool of gastric juice* to avoid reflux or aspiration during the procedure

5 *insufflate the stomach* enough to obtain a reasonable view during insertion

6 *inject a suspension of silicone* (simethicone) down the biopsy channel if there is excessive foaming. If this is used, it must be flushed completely out of the scope before reprocessing.

The four walls of the stomach are examined sequentially by a combination of tip deflection, instrument rotation and advancement/withdrawal. It is important to be both systematic and deliberate so as to minimize the amount of unexamined surface area. The field of view during the advance of a four-way angling endoscope can be represented as a cylinder angulated over the vertebral bodies. The distended stomach takes up an exaggerated J-shape with the axis of the advancing instrument corkscrewing clockwise up and over the spine, following the greater curvature (Fig 5.14). Limiting insufflation during endoscope advancement into the stomach can help reduce the insertion route and time by shortening the stomach's longitudinal axis.

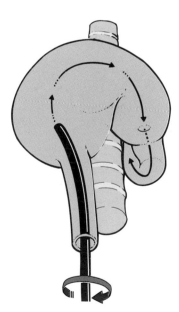

Fig 5.14 The route to pylorus and duodenum is a clockwise spiral around the vertebral column.

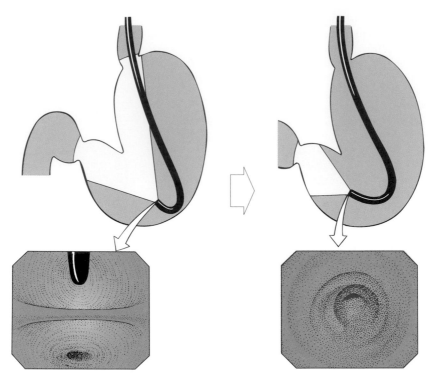

Fig 5.15 The angulus and antrum come into view . . .

Fig 5.16 . . . then angle down to see the pylorus in the axis of the antrum.

Thus, to advance through the stomach and into the antrum:

1 *angle the tip up (toward 12 o'clock) increasingly*
2 *rotate the shaft clockwise ("turn right")*.

This clockwise corkscrew rotation through approximately 90° during insertion brings the angulus and antrum into end-on view (Fig 5.15). Clockwise torque can be achieved by moving the left hand/arm from a horizontal to vertical (upright) position. It may be necessary now to deflect the tip a little downward to bring it into the axis of the antrum (Fig 5.16), so that it runs smoothly along its greater curve and the tip is angled toward the pylorus. The motor activity of the antrum, pyloric canal, and pyloric ring should be carefully observed. Asymmetry during a peristaltic wave is a useful indicator of present or previous disease.

Through the pylorus into the duodenum

The pyloric ring is approached directly for passage into the duodenum. During the maneuver it is convenient to use only the left hand for tip angulation and torque to maintain the instrument tip in the correct axis.

1 *Advance with the pyloric ring in the center of the view*.
2 Intubate the duodenal bulb by advancing the scope as close as possible to the pyloric ring and then *apply gentle pressure*; insufflation may also be helpful. Passage is both felt and seen. Entry into

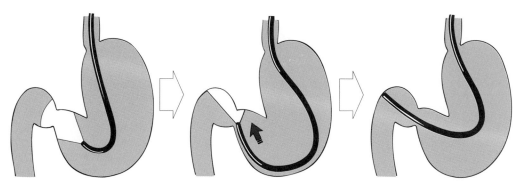

Fig 5.17 The scope passes from the antrum . . .

Fig 5.18 . . . to the pylorus and duodenal cap . . .

Fig 5.19 . . . and tends to impact in the duodenum.

the duodenal bulb is recognized by its granular and pale surface (Figs 5.17, 5.18, and 5.19).

3 Patience may be needed to pass the pylorus, especially if there is spasm or deformity; ***downward*** angulation of the tip or deflation may help its passage. As the instrument tip passes the resistance of the pylorus, the loop that has inevitably developed in the stomach straightens out and may accelerate the tip to the distal bulb (Fig 5.19).

4 So, to obtain optimal views of the duodenal bulb, ***withdraw a few centimeters to disimpact the tip and insufflate*** (Fig 5.20).

5 ***Examine the bulb by circumferential manipulation of the tip*** during endoscope advancement and withdrawal. The area immediately beyond the pyloric ring, especially the inferior part of the bulb, may be missed by the inexperienced, who fail to withdraw sufficiently for fear of falling back into the stomach.

6 ***Give an antispasmodic*** (Buscopan® or glucagon) intravenously if visualization is impaired by duodenal motility.

7 ***Avoid excessive insufflation***, which will leave the patient uncomfortably distended.

Passage into the descending duodenum

The superior duodenal angle is the key landmark (Fig 5.20) connecting the bulb and the descending duodenum. To pass into the descending duodenum, ***gently***:

1 ***advance so that the tip lies at the angle***

2 ***rotate the shaft about 90° clockwise ("turn right")***, by either applying rotation to the endoscope shaft with the right hand, bringing the left hand (which holds the endoscope head) in toward the chest, and/or turning the body to the right.

3 ***simultaneously deflect the tip up.***

This maneuver creates a corkscrew motion around the angle (Fig 5.21) and provides a tunnel view of the descending (second portion) duodenum with its typical circular folds (valves of Kerckring). To advance further ***do not just push***, which will simply form a big loop in the stomach (Fig 5.22). Rather, it is necessary to ***pull back***. This paradoxical maneuver straightens the loop in the stomach propelling the tip onward, and the

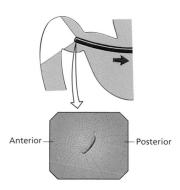

Anterior — — Posterior

Fig 5.20 Withdraw the scope to disimpact the tip and insufflate to see the superior duodenal angle—an important landmark.

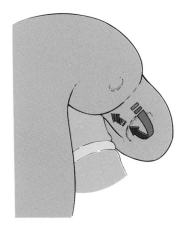

Fig 5.21 Corkscrew the tip clockwise around the superior duodenal angle, using clockwise torque, and right angulation simultaneously.

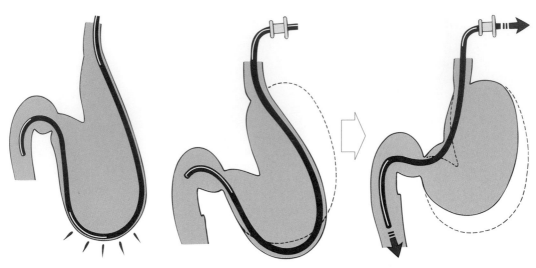

Fig 5.22 Trying to reach the third part by force simply forms a loop in the stomach.

Fig 5.23 . . . withdrawal helps to advance the scope into the second part of the duodenum.

Fig 5.24 Because of the loop in the greater curve . . .

straightening shaft corkscrews the tip round the superior duodenal angle (Figs 5.23 and 5.24). Using the correct "pull and twist" method, the tip slides in to reach the region of the major papilla with only about 60 cm of instrument inserted. A forward-viewing instrument gives tangential and often restricted views of the convex medial wall of the descending duodenum and the papilla. Much better views of this area are obtained with side-viewing instruments.

Withdrawal back into the stomach

The mucosa is usually inspected in greater detail during the withdrawal phase. To withdraw the endoscope from the duodenum, the opposite movements are required, including pull back, counterclockwise rotation and downward tip deflection. Care should be taken to withdraw slowly along the duodenal sweep as the endoscope tends to fall out quickly and lesions may be missed.

Retroflexion in the stomach (J maneuver) and U-turn maneuver

The fundus of the stomach is often best seen in retroversion (i.e. from below) to ensure that blind spots are visualized. To achieve this view safely:

1 *place the tip of the endoscope in the mid stomach*, at or just beyond the angulus (gastric angle) such that the distal antrum and pyloric ring are visualized

2 *insufflate air*

3 *simultaneously advance the scope and angle the endoscope tip up acutely 180°* into a J-shape (using both angulation control knobs); this "J maneuver" should demonstrate the angulus, the entire lesser curve, and the fundus as the instrument is withdrawn (Fig 5.25)

4 *pull back slowly* to move the tip into the fundus; *do not pull back too far*, as this risks impacting the retroverted tip in the distal esophagus

5 *rotate the shaft in both directions (U-turn or "missed clap" maneuver)* to obtain complete 360° views of the fundus and cardia (Fig 5.26); rotating the right/left angulation control knob to the maximal extent in both directions can aid in viewing the cardia

6 *after retroversion, remember to return the angulation controls to the neutral position.*

Retroflexion in the stomach is probably best performed after examining the duodenum so as to avoid overinflation on the way in. Some patients (particularly those with a lax cardia) find it difficult to hold enough CO_2/air to permit an adequate view. If retroversion proves difficult, it may be made easier by rotating the patient slightly onto their back to give the stomach more room to expand.

During all of these maneuvers, it is helpful to keep the shaft of the instrument relatively straight from the patient's teeth to your hands. This reduces the strain on the endoscope, helps orientation, and ensures that your rotating movements are precisely transmitted to the tip.

Removing the instrument

The mucosa should be surveyed carefully once again during withdrawal, using tip deflection and torque to view the stomach. Under the different motility conditions and organ shapes produced by distension and instrument position, areas previously seen only tangentially on insertion may be brought into direct view on the way out. The proximal lesser curve, a potential "blind spot," merits particular attention as the scope withdraws along it. Remember to aspirate CO_2/air (and fluid) from the stomach completely on withdrawal, and to release the brakes from the angulation controls (if they have been applied). Take a moment to measure the level of the gastroesophageal junction. Then withdraw the instrument up through the esophagus, adjusting the hand to maintain the grip at a consistent distance (Video 5.2).

Finally, take a few seconds to reassure the patient, "Well done, it's all over, we will talk in a few minutes. . . ."

Now begin the cleaning process! It is important not to let blood and secretions dry on the instrument or in the channels. So, immediately:

1 *wipe the endoscope with a wet cloth*

2 *place the tip in water and depress both control valves* (to flush out any mucus or blood from the air/water channel and wash through the instrumentation channel)

3 *hand the instrument to the nurse/assistant* to start the cleaning and disinfection process.

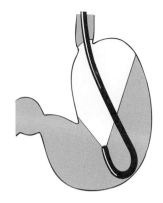

Fig 5.25 Angulation of 180° (J maneuver) retroflexes the tip to see the lesser curve . . .

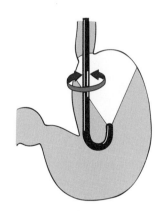

Fig 5.26 . . . and rotation of retroflexed tip (U-turn) in both directions provides a 360° view of the fundus and cardia.

Problems during endoscopy

Patient distress

Endoscopy should be terminated quickly if the patient shows distress for which the cause is not immediately obvious and remediable. If reassurance does not calm the patient, remove the instrument and consider giving additional sedation or analgesia. Inadvertent bronchoscopy can occur if insertion is done by the "blind" method, and it is obvious from the unusual view and impressive coughing. Discomfort may arise from inappropriate pressure during intubation or from distension due to excessive insufflation. Remember to keep inflation to a minimum and to aspirate all the CO_2/air at the end of the procedure. Severe pain during endoscopy is very rare and indicates an adverse event such as perforation or a cardiac incident. It is extremely dangerous to ignore warning signs. Tachycardia and bradycardia may both indicate distress.

Getting lost

The endoscopist may become disoriented and the instrument looped in patients with congenital malrotations or major pathology (e.g. achalasia, large diverticula, hernias) or after complex surgery. Careful study of any available radiographs may help. The most common reason for disorientation in patients with normal anatomy is inadequate insufflation due to a defect in the instrument, CO_2 insufflator or air pump (which should have been detected before starting the examination). Inexperienced endoscopists often get lost in the fundus, especially when the stomach is angled acutely over the vertebral column. Having passed the cardia, the instrument tip should be deflected to the endoscopist's *left* (counterclockwise) and slightly downward (Fig 5.27). A wrong turn to the right (clockwise) will bring the tip back up into the fundus. When in doubt, withdraw, insufflate, and turn sharply left (counterclockwise) to find the true lumen. A curious endoscopic view may indicate perforation (which is not always immediately painful). If a visible perforation is detected (presence of a hole, protrusion of yellow peritoneal fat, or a view of peritoneal organs), there are some immediate therapeutic interventions that may be employed by an experienced, advanced endoscopist to close the defect, including over-the-scope metal clips and endoscopic suturing. When such expertise is not readily available, or if no hole is seen but there remains any doubt about a possible perforation, abandon the examination and obtain radiological studies.

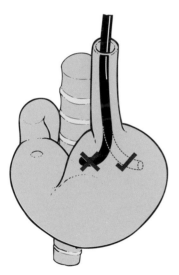

Fig 5.27 Angling right (rather than left) on entering the fundus can cause retroflexion and can result in getting lost.

Inadequate mucosal view

Lack of a clear view means that the lens is lying against the mucosa or is obscured by fluid or food debris. Withdraw slightly and insufflate; double check that the CO_2/air pump is working and that all connections are firm with O-rings present. Try washing the lens with the normal finger-controlled water jet. This may not be effective if the instrument lens is covered by debris (or by mucosa that has been sucked onto the orifice of the biopsy channel). Pressure can be released by brief removal of the rubber valve of the biopsy port, but it may be necessary to flush the channel with water or air using a syringe. Small quantities of food or mucus obscuring an area of interest can be washed away with a jet of water. Foaming can be suppressed by adding a diluted emulsion of silicone (simethicone).

As most patients comply with instructions to fast before procedures, the presence of excessive food residue is an important sign of outlet obstruction or gastroparesis. Standard endoscope channels are too small for aspiration of food; prolonged attempts simply result in blocked channels. The instrument can usually be guided along the lesser curvature over the top of the food to allow a search for a distal obstructing lesion. The greater curvature can also be examined, if necessary, by rotating the patient into the right lateral position. However, any examination in the presence of excess fluid or food carries a significant risk of regurgitation and pulmonary aspiration so airway protection via an endotracheal tube is recommended. The endoscopist should persist only if the immediate benefits are thought to justify the risk. It is usually wiser to stop and to repeat the examination only after proper gastric lavage.

Recognition of lesions

This book is concerned mainly with techniques, rather than with lesions. Several excellent atlases are available. However, certain points are worth emphasizing here.

Esophagus
Esophagitis

Esophagitis normally follows acid reflux and is most apparent distally, close to the gastroesophageal mucosal junction. If the distal esophagus is normal with areas of inflammation in the mid or proximal esophagus, the cause is probably not due to reflux (drug or viral causes). The earliest visible reflux changes consist of mucosal congestion and edema that obscure the normal fine vascular pattern, progressing to short breaks in the surface of the longitudinal esophageal folds (Fig 5.28), leading in more severe grades (Los Angeles classification) to longer linear breaks, then damage that is confluent or extends circumferentially. The process culminates in symmetrical stricturing, above which the mucosa (now protected from reflux) may appear almost normal.

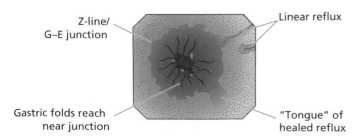

Fig 5.28 Minor reflux changes above hiatus hernia—no need for biopsies.

Eosinophilic esophagitis

Endoscopy and mucosal biopsies play an important role in the diagnosis and management of eosinophilic esophagitis. A total of six biopsies should be taken from at least two levels of the esophagus. Several endoscopic findings are associated with eosinophilic esophagitis, including edema (decreased mucosal vascularity or pallor), rings (trachealization), exudate (white spots or plaques), longitudinal furrows, esophageal strictures, narrow caliber esophagus, and crepe paper esophagus (mucosal fragility).

Barrett's esophagus

Barrett's esophagus is a potentially precancerous consequence of longstanding reflux damage. Red gastric-type mucosa is seen endoscopically to extend proximally from the top of the gastric folds in a semi-inflated esophagus. The pattern of this columnar extension may be in "tongues" or "circumferential" (or both), sometimes with columnar "islands" proximal to that. The maximum extent (in centimeters) of tongues or circumferential change should each be recorded (Prague classification). Quadrantic biopsies are taken every 2 cm circumferentially and from tongues or islands, looking for "specialized intestinal metaplasia" (Barrett's epithelium) and for any dysplasia within it (Fig 5.29). As long as no dysplasia is present, surveillance endoscopies can be performed every 2–5 years. Mucosal dysplasia in Barrett's and elsewhere in the GI tract is characterized by abrupt changes from the background surrounding tissue in color (often with sharp demarcation), loss of the regular mucosal pattern, localized nodularity and/or depression, and prominent irregularly shaped and thickened blood vessel patterns.

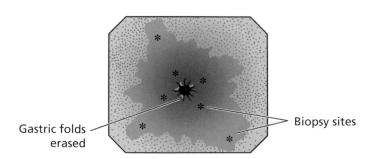

Gastric folds erased   Biopsy sites

Fig 5.29 Barrett's esophagus—take biopsies.

Esophageal carcinoma

Esophageal carcinoma usually causes asymmetrical stenosis, with areas of exuberant abnormal mucosa and sometimes an irregular ulcer with raised edges. Carcinoma of the gastric fundus may also infiltrate upward submucosally to involve the esophagus. The correct diagnosis is then easily made if the endoscope can be passed through the stricture to allow retroverted views of the cardia. However, superficial flat early squamous cancers may occur and appear only as localized blemishes that reveal abnormal blood vessels on closer inspection.

Diverticula

Diverticula in the mid- or distal esophagus are easily recognized, but the instrument may enter a pulsion diverticulum (Zenker's) or pouch in the upper esophagus without the true lumen being seen at all. Lack of view and resistance to inward movement are (as always) an indication to pull back and reassess. Diverticula found in the mid-esophagus are caused by inflammatory swelling and subsequent contraction of subcarinal lymph nodes. These are termed "traction diverticula." Webs or rings, such as the Schatzki ring, at or just proximal to the gastroesophageal junction may not be obvious to the endoscopist because of a combination of "flat" bright endoscope illumination and distortion from the wide-angled lens view.

Varices

Varices lie in the long axis of the esophagus as tortuous bluish mounds covered with relatively normal mucosa. They resemble varicose veins elsewhere in the body.

Mallory-Weiss tears

Mallory-Weiss tears are 5–20 mm longitudinal mucosal splits lying on either side of or across the gastroesophageal mucosal junction. These are thought to be caused by retching, but a history of this can be elicited in only 50% of cases. In the acute phase the tear is covered with exudate or clot and may sometimes be seen best in a retroverted view.

Motility disturbances

Motility disturbances of the esophagus should be diagnosed by radiology and manometry, but their consequences—such as dilation, pseudodiverticula, food retention, and esophagitis—are well seen at endoscopy, which is usually needed to rule out obstructing pathology.

Achalasia typically appears as a dilated, fluid-filled esophagus with ineffective or absent peristalsis. The endoscope passes easily through the lower esophageal sphincter and into the cardia, in contrast to the fixed narrowing of pathological strictures due to reflux esophagitis or malignancy.

Stomach

The appearance of the normal gastric mucosa varies considerably. Reddening (hyperemia) may be generalized (e.g. with bile reflux into the operated stomach) or localized. Sometimes it occurs in long streaks along the ridges of mucosal folds. Localized (traumatic) reddening with or without petechiae or edematous changes is often seen on the posterior upper lesser curve in patients who habitually retch. Macroscopic congestion does not correlate well with underlying histological gastritis, and care should be taken when considering clinical relevance. Biopsy samples should be taken when any abnormality is suspected, and tests for *Helicobacter pylori* performed in patients with dyspepsia with or without macroscopic lesions.

Gastric folds

Gastric folds vary in size, but the endoscopic assessment also depends upon the degree of gastric distension. Very prominent fleshy folds are seen in Ménétrier's disease and are best diagnosed by a snare-loop biopsy. Patients with duodenal ulceration often have large gastric folds with spotty areas of congestion within the areae gastricae and excess quantities of clear resting juice. With gastric atrophy, there are no mucosal folds (when the stomach is distended) and blood vessels are easily seen through the pale atrophic mucosa. Atrophy is often associated with intestinal metaplasia, which appears as small, gray-white plaques.

Erosions and ulcers

Erosions and ulcers are the most common localized gastric lesions. A lesion is usually called an erosion if it is small (<5 mm diameter) and shallow, with no sign of scarring. Acute ulcers and erosions are often seen in the antrum and may be capped with, and partially obscured by, clots. Edematous erosions appear as small, smooth, umbilicated raised areas, often in chains along the folds of the gastric body. "Gastritis" is a term best reserved for histological use.

The classic chronic benign gastric ulcer is usually single and is most frequently seen on the lesser curvature at or above the angulus. It is typically symmetrical with smooth margins and a clean base (unless there are eroding adjacent structures). Multiple and punched out ulcers (sometimes oddly shaped and very large) occur in some patients taking nonsteroidal anti-inflammatory drugs (NSAIDs).

Malignancy

Malignancy may be suspected if an ulcer has raised irregular margins (or different heights around the circumference), a lumpy hemorrhagic base or a mucosal abnormality surrounding the ulcer. Mucosal folds around a benign ulcer usually radiate toward it and reach the margin. At times it may be difficult to separate benign from malignant ulcers on macroscopic appearance alone; if there is doubt, tissue specimens should be taken from the ulcer edge. Unfortunately, gastric cancer is usually diagnosed at an advanced stage in Western countries, when it is all too obvious at endoscopy. Diffusely infiltrating carcinoma (*linitis plastica*) may be missed unless motility is carefully studied. Standard mucosal biopsies may be normal, and a high degree of suspicion is required. Endoscopic ultrasonography (EUS) is the best method of differentiating the cause of enlarged gastric folds.

Early gastric cancers may mimic a small benign ulcer, chronic erosion, or a flat polyp. They may also appear only as a well-demarcated but flat area of redness in which, on closer inspection, the usual mucosal pattern of the surrounding mucosa is abruptly lost. For this reason, small, localized areas of altered color, especially with discrete edges, need to be recognized and examined closely.

Polypoid lesions under 1 cm in diameter are usually benign in origin. However, as all malignant lesions start small and are curable if detected at an early stage, odd mucosal lumps and bumps should never be ignored; a tissue diagnosis must be made. Submucosal tumors are characterized by normal overlying mucosa and bridging folds; leiomyomas and plaques of aberrant pancreatic tissue (characteristically found in the floor of the antrum) usually have a central dimple or crater.

Duodenum
Duodenal ulcers
Duodenal ulcers, either current or previous, often cause persistent deformity of the duodenal bulb and/or pyloric ring. The ulcers occur most commonly on the anterior and posterior walls of the bulb and are frequently multiple. When active, they are surrounded by edema and acute congestion. Scarring often results in a characteristic shelf-like deformity, which partially divides the bulb and may produce a pseudodiverticulum. A small linear ulcer or scar can be seen running along the apex of this fold. The mucosa of the bulb often reveals small mucosal changes of dubious clinical significance. Areas of mucosal congestion with spotty white exudate ("pepper and salt" ulceration) merge into even less definite macroscopic appearances labeled as "duodenitis." Small mucosal lumps in the proximal duodenum usually reflect underlying Brunner's gland hyperplasia or gastric metaplasia (ectopic islands of gastric mucosa). Duodenal tumors occur mainly in the region of the papilla of Vater.

Ulceration and duodenitis in the second part of the duodenum suggests Zollinger-Ellison syndrome or underlying pancreatic disease. Crohn's disease may be suspected by the presence of small aphthous ulcers in the second part; typical granulomas may be seen on histology.

Celiac disease
Celiac disease is now known to be significantly more common than previously thought. The characteristic finding is "scalloping" of the small bowel folds, which represent defects (bites) in the mucosa. Other common endoscopic features of celiac disease comprise a mosaic appearance, nodularity and a reduction or loss of circular duodenal folds. A useful "trick" is to fill the second/third portion of the duodenum with water. Water magnifies the endoscopic image. In normal cases, small villi will be easily seen swaying back and forth under water. If the villi are blunted, diminished, or absent, celiac disease should be suspected, and biopsies should be obtained from both the duodenal cap (one to two biopsies) and the distal portion of the duodenum (four biopsies).

Dye enhancement techniques
Dye enhancement techniques may assist the recognition of inconspicuous mucosal lesions such as those found in celiac disease. Dye spraying (chromoscopy) is best achieved by spraying with a tube and fine nozzle applied close to the mucosa. The dye fills the interstices, highlighting irregularities in architecture. Indigo carmine is used most commonly. Intravital staining is an alternative approach

to lesion enhancement. Stains such as methylene blue, Lugol's solution, and toluidine blue may be taken up preferentially in diseased mucosa (such as intestinal metaplasia). Fluorescent stains (given intravenously) may highlight lesions under special conditions such as ultraviolet illumination. Optical techniques such as narrow band imaging (NBI), Fuji Intelligent Chromo Endoscopy (FICE), and iScan may offer similar benefit for identifying mucosal lesions without the need for dye.

Specimen collection

Many factors determine the diagnostic yield of tissue sampling, including adequacy of the specimens, handling, processing, and interpretation. It is important to emphasize the need for close collaboration between endoscopy and laboratory staff. The diagnostic yield from endoscopic specimens will be maximized if laboratory staff are involved in defining the methods for specimen handling and transmission. Specimens should reach the laboratory with precise details of their origin and the specific clinical question that needs to be answered. Pathologists who routinely receive a copy of the endoscopy findings (and later follow-up) are more likely to give timely and relevant reports. Regular review sessions should be part of the quality improvement process.

Biopsy techniques

The number and location of biopsies obtained will vary based on procedural indication and findings. Biopsy specimens are taken with cupped forceps. The lesion should be approached face-on, so that firm and direct pressure can be applied to it with the widely opened cups. Pressure is easier to apply if the forceps are kept close to the endoscope tip. Better control is achieved by advancing the scope to the target rather than the forceps. Similarly, specimens from the esophagus are best taken by angling the tip of the endoscope acutely against the wall and positioning the forceps such that they are *en face* to the mucosa and barely protruding. The forceps are closed gently but firmly by an assistant when directed to grab the tissue and then snapped back into the endoscope. Forceps with a central spike between opposing biopsy cups generally obtain deeper biopsies and make it easier to take specimens from lesions that have to be approached tangentially (e.g. in the esophagus). Spiked forceps, sometimes termed double-bite forceps, may also allow for two specimens to be taken before withdrawing the forceps, as the spike acts to hold the first biopsy while the second is obtained. Some experts prefer not to use spiked forceps because of the risk of accidental skin puncture. Multi-bite forceps enable consecutive acquisition of up to four or more tissue specimens with a single pass through the accessory channel, potentially decreasing overall procedure time when many specimens need to be obtained (e.g. colon cancer surveillance in patients with longstanding inflammatory bowel disease).

Ulcer biopsies should be taken from the ulcer rim in all four quadrants; basal specimens may be taken if a viral process is suspected, but for other entities they usually yield only slough. When sampling proliferative tumors it is wise to avoid necrotic areas, as they often produce nondiagnostic specimens.

The methods for handling and fixing specimens should be established after discussion with the relevant pathologist. Some prefer samples to be gently flattened on paper or other surfaces such as cellulose filter (Millipore, etc.). The cellulose filter method of biopsy mounting has considerable advantages for the management of multiple small endoscopic biopsies: they adhere well to the filter and are rarely lost; they are mounted in sequence so that errors of location are impossible; and they allow the histopathologist to view serial sections of six to eight biopsies at a time in a row across a single microscope slide. A 15 mm strip of cellulose filter (just less than the width of a glass slide) has a pencil-ruled or printed central line and a notch or mark made at one end (Fig 5.30a). Each biopsy is eased out of the forceps cup with the tip of a micropipette or toothpick (to avoid needle-stick injuries) (Fig 5.30b), placed exactly onto the line and patted flat (Fig 5.30c). The strip with its line of biopsies is placed into fixative (Fig 5.30d). In the laboratory it is processed, wax-mounted in the correct orientation (Fig 5.30e), sectioned through the line of biopsies on the filter (Fig 5.30f), positioned on the microscope slide (Fig 5.30g), and then stained and examined without

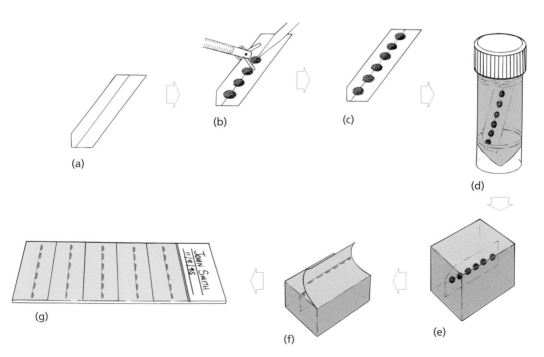

Fig 5.30 Stages in placing biopsies onto the filter then fixing, sectioning, and mounting the specimens.

handling the biopsies individually at any stage. A dissecting microscope or hand lens can be used to orientate mucosal specimens before fixation if information is required about the mucosal architecture (e.g. duodenal biopsies in malabsorption).

If detection of *H. pylori* infection is important, at least two biopsy specimens should be taken from the gastric antrum, two from the middle of the body, and consider one from the incisura. The specimen requisition should specifically state if *H. pylori* is suspected, as some pathology labs will not routinely do additional stains for *H. pylori* on gastric biopsies.

Biopsy sites often bleed trivially but sometimes sufficiently to obscure the lesion before adequate samples have been taken. For this reason, detailed mucosal inspection for possible abnormalities should precede collection of biopsy samples. If visualization is obscured, the area should be washed with a jet of water or a 1:100,000 solution of epinephrine (adrenaline). Bleeding of clinical significance is exceptionally rare.

Cytology techniques

Cytology specimens are taken under direct vision with a sleeved brush (Fig 5.31), which is passed through the instrument channel. The head of the brush is advanced out of its sleeve and rubbed and rolled repeatedly across the surface of the lesion; a circumferential sweep of the margin and base of an ulcer is desirable. The brush is then pulled back into the sleeve, and both are withdrawn together. The brush is protruded, wiped over two or three glass slides and then rapidly fixed before drying damages the cells. The precise method of preparation (in the unit or laboratory) should be determined by the cytologist. Brushes should not be reused. A trap (Fig 5.32) can be used to collect cytology specimens. Suction through the channel after a biopsy procedure ("salvage cytology") also produces useful cellular material.

The value of brush cytology depends largely on the skill and enthusiasm of the cytopathologist. Many studies indicate that a combination of brush cytology and biopsy provides a higher yield than biopsy alone. In practice most endoscopists reserve cytology for lesions from which good biopsy specimens are difficult to obtain (e.g. tight esophageal strictures) and for resampling a suspicious lesion. It is also commonly used for collecting samples for suspected candida esophagitis. Taking aspiration samples for cytology through a needle may occasionally be useful.

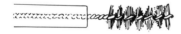

Fig 5.31 Cytology brush with outer sleeve.

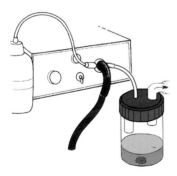

Fig 5.32 A suction trap to collect fluid specimens.

Sampling submucosal lesions

Standard biopsy specimens are usually normal in patients with submucosal lesions (such as benign tumors), as the forceps do not traverse the muscularis mucosae. One exception is carcinoid tumors. These often originate from the deep mucosa and can usually be diagnosed from standard biopsy specimens. Larger and deeper specimens can be taken with a diathermy snare loop, as described with polypectomy in Chapter 8.

An alternative method for obtaining deeper tissue samples is to use a needle to obtain samples for cytology. EUS-guided fine needle aspiration is increasingly popular in this context.

Diagnostic endoscopy under special circumstances

Operated patients

Unless prevented by postoperative stenosis, endoscopy is the best method for diagnosis and exclusion of mucosal inflammation, recurrent ulcers, and tumors after upper gastrointestinal surgery. The endoscopist can document the size and arrangement of any outlet or anastomosis, but barium radiology and nuclear medicine techniques may be needed to give more information about motility and emptying disorders.

Experience is needed to appreciate the wide range of "normal" endoscopic appearance in the operated patient. Postoperative anatomy may be difficult to identify, particularly if there are multiple efferent lumens. Partial gastrectomy, gastroenterostomy, and pyloroplasty result in reflux of bile and intestinal juice. Resultant foaming in the stomach may obscure the endoscopic view and should be suppressed by flushing with a silicone suspension. Gastric distension is difficult to maintain in patients with a large gastric outlet; avoid pumping too much air and overdistending the intestine. Most patients who have undergone partial gastrectomy or gastroenterostomy have impressively hyperemic mucosae. Initially this is most marked close to the stoma, but atrophic gastritis is progressive, and plaques of grayish-white intestinal metaplasia may be seen. There is an increased risk of cancer in the gastric remnant, particularly close to the stoma. Cancers in this site can be difficult to recognize endoscopically. If the clinical suspicion for malignancy is high, multiple biopsy specimens from within 3 cm of the stoma should be taken.

Ulcers following partial gastrectomy or gastroenterostomy usually occur at or just beyond the anastomosis. Endoscopic diagnosis is usually simple, but the area just beneath the stoma may sometimes be difficult to survey completely using a forward-viewing instrument. A lateral-viewing endoscope may also sometimes allow a more complete survey in a scarred and tortuous pyloroplasty. Many surgeons use nonabsorbable sutures when performing an intestinal anastomosis; these can ulcerate through the mucosa and appear as black or green threads and loops. Their clinical significance remains controversial. Endoscopy is occasionally performed (for bleeding or stomal obstruction) within a few days of upper gastrointestinal tract surgery. In these cases air insufflation should be kept to a minimum.

Acute upper gastrointestinal bleeding

Bleeding provides special challenges for the endoscopist, and details are given in Chapter 6.

Endoscopy in children

Ensuring safe and effective endoscopy in children requires adequate knowledge and skills specific to performing pediatric endoscopic procedures. Procedures in children should ideally be performed by an individual with training in pediatric endoscopy. When adult endoscopists perform pediatric procedures, collaboration with a pediatric specialist is warranted.

Pediatric endoscopy is not just a matter of size; there are differences related to the procedure itself as well as the patients, including age-related physiology, informed consent processes, and differing indications and spectrum of disease in children. A key difference between pediatric and adult diagnostic upper endoscopy is that routine tissue sampling is performed in children from at least the duodenum, stomach, and esophagus even in the absence of macroscopic findings.

A child-friendly and family-centered setting with appropriate equipment is also necessary. Gastroscope type should depend on the child's weight and age. The standard adult forward- and lateral-viewing instruments (8–11 mm diameter) can be used in children greater than 10 kg or 1 year of age. An ultra-slim pediatric gastroscope (≤6 mm diameter) is preferred for infants under 10 kg or a year of age. Some ultrathin gastroscopes only have two-way (up/down) tip deflection and are dependent on application of torque for right/left visualization. An adult gastroscope can be considered in children >5 kg if endotherapy is required, as the small operating channel of pediatric gastroscopes (1.5–2 mm) decreases suctioning capabilities and limits the range of possible therapeutic options, as not all endoscopic devices are produced for ultra-slim endoscopes.

Upper endoscopy in children is suggested to be performed under general anesthesia or, only if general anesthesia is not available, under deep sedation in a carefully monitored environment. In general, anesthetic sedation levels requiring endotracheal intubation are not needed for routine diagnostic endoscopy, but rather for therapeutic interventions or complex patients. There is a risk of excessive insufflation when using anesthesia or deep sedation in the smallest children; CO_2 for insufflation is preferable and it is wise to keep the abdomen exposed during examination and to palpate it regularly. Careful monitoring of oxygenation and the pulse is essential and pediatric-specific monitoring and resuscitation equipment must be available, as children can have sudden and severe reactions to sedative agents.

Endoscopy of the small intestine

Visualizing most or all of the small intestine is a challenge, but significant advances have been made in recent years. The third and fourth parts of the duodenum can usually be examined with standard forward-viewing endoscopes. This is often best achieved (as with colonoscopy) by pulling back to straighten the scope, deflating the stomach, applying abdominal pressure and maybe changing the patient's position.

Deep enteroscopy. Longer and more flexible endoscopes ("enteroscopes") can be pushed into the upper jejunum, but deeper insertion requires adjuvant devices. The simplest is a stiffening overtube, which prevents bowing in the stomach. Better results are now obtained with balloon-assisted enteroscopy and spiral enteroscopy. Enteroscopes with sleeves and one or two inflatable balloons allow skilled endoscopists to navigate large portions of the small bowel. The balloon acts as an intermittent "tether" as the scope is repeatedly straightened, then advanced. The same type of instrument can be used though the anus, to allow ileoscopy from below. Spiral enteroscopy involves a sleeve with a "corkscrew" device and has similar yield to balloon-assisted enteroscopy. Despite these developments, the extent of mucosal examination is variable and unpredictable. The procedure does cause some mucosal artifacts, which may mimic erosions.

Capsule endoscopy is a paradigm shift in digestive endoscopy and is a remarkable technical achievement. Essentially the patient swallows a small camera (about the size of a Brazil nut), which transmits images to an external receiver. The images are examined at leisure. While automated lesion-detection solutions are commercially available, further prospective studies are required before they can be applied in clinical practice and interpretation should be by a trained endoscopist. This technique has become popular for examining patients with gastrointestinal bleeding that is unexplained after standard procedures, evaluation of Crohn's disease, and for surveillance in patients with a polyposis syndrome. Its use is being extended into screening the esophagus and even the colon. The capsule does not currently have any therapeutic potential, so lesions, when found, often must be sought again and treated by deep enteroscopy or surgery.

Further reading

ASGE Training Committee, Kwon RS, Davila RE, et al. EGD core curriculum. *Gastrointest Endosc* 2017;2(7):162–8.

Bisschops R, Areia M, Coron E, et al. Performance measures for upper gastrointestinal endoscopy: A European Society of Gastrointestinal Endoscopy (ESGE) quality improvement initiative. *Endoscopy* 2016; 48(9):843–64.

Cohen J. *Comprehensive Atlas of High-Resolution Endoscopy and Narrowband Imaging* (2nd edition). Chichester, United Kingdom: Wiley Blackwell, 2017.

Coronel E, Waxman I. Upper gastrointestinal endoscopy. In: Wang TC, Camilleri M, eds. *Yamada's Atlas of Gastroenterology* (6th edition). Hoboken, NJ: John Wiley & Sons, 2022:687–712.

Enns RA, Hookey L, Armstrong A, et al. Clinical practice guidelines for the use of video capsule endoscopy. *Gastroenterology* 2017;152(3): 497–514.

Hirota WK, Zuckerman MJ, Adler DG, et al. ASGE guideline: The role of endoscopy in the surveillance of premalignant conditions of the upper gastrointestinal tract. *Gastrointest Endosc* 2006;63(4):570–80.

Lightdale JR, Walsh CM, Oliva S, et al. Pediatric Endoscopy Quality Improvement Network quality standards and indicators for pediatric endoscopic procedures: A joint NASPGHAN/ESPGHAN guideline. *J Pediatr Gastroenterol Nutr* 2022;74(S1 Suppl 1):S30–S43.

Melson J, Trikudanathan G, Abu Dayyeh BK, et al. Video capsule endoscopy. *Gastrointest Endosc* 2021;93(4):784–96.

Park WG, Shaheen NJ, Cohen J, et al. Quality indicators for EGD. *Gastrointest Endosc* 2015;81(1):17–30.

Sidhu R, Sanders DS, Morris AJ, McAlindon ME. Guidelines on small bowel enteroscopy and capsule endoscopy in adults. *Gut* 2008;57(1):125–36.

Sidhu R, Zammit SC, Baltes P, et al. Curriculum for small-bowel capsule endoscopy and device-assisted enteroscopy training in Europe: European Society of Gastrointestinal Endoscopy (ESGE) Position Statement. *Endoscopy* 2020;52(8):669–86.

Tringali A, Thomson M, Dumonceau J-M, et al. Pediatric gastrointestinal endoscopy: European Society of Gastrointestinal Endoscopy (ESGE) and European Society for Paediatric Gastroenterology Hepatology and Nutrition (ESPGHAN) guideline executive summary. *Endoscopy* 2017;49(1):83–91.

Walsh CM, Lightdale JR, Mack DR, et al. Overview of the Pediatric Endoscopy Quality Improvement Network quality standards and indicators for pediatric endoscopy: A joint NASPGHAN/ESPGHAN guideline. *J Pediatr Gastroenterol Nutr* 2022;74(S1 Suppl 1):S3–S15.

Chapter video clips (www.wiley.com/go/cottonwilliams8e)

Video 5.1 Endoscopic view of direct vision insertion
Video 5.2 Full insertion and examination

CHAPTER 6

Therapeutic Upper Endoscopy

Today's gastroenterologists have a major role in the interventional treatment of many upper gastrointestinal problems. Established techniques include the management of dysphagia (due to benign and malignant esophageal stenoses and achalasia), polyps, gastric and duodenal stenoses, foreign bodies, acute bleeding, and nutritional support. Other innovative therapies, such as the endoscopic treatment of reflux, and of obesity, are emerging.

Benign esophageal strictures

Gastroesophageal reflux is the commonest cause of benign esophageal strictures. Other causes include eosinophilic esophagitis, fungal and viral infections, medications, caustic ingestion, extrinsic compression, and therapeutic interventions (surgery, endoscopy, and radiation).

In general, dysphagia occurs when a stricture causes greater than 50% of the esophageal lumen to be obstructed or the esophageal lumen is less than about 13 mm. It follows that easy passage of a standard endoscope (8–10 mm diameter) does not exclude a problem, or the possible need for treatment.

Dilation methods

Dilation is used only as part of an overall treatment plan, with due attention also to diet, lifestyle modification, and necessary medications. Surgery is needed in a few recalcitrant cases.

Even though there are many dilation techniques and varieties of equipment, they fall into two main categories: *mechanical* (push-type or bougie) or *balloon* dilators. While the exact mechanism is not clear, the mechanical dilators exert a longitudinal and radial force, dilating proximal to distal on the stricture, opposed to the purely radial force delivered simultaneously across the stricture by the balloon dilators (Fig 6.1).

To ensure correct placement, dilating balloons or graduated wire-guided bougies, under endoscopic and/or fluoroscopic control (over a guidewire), are preferred for dilation to ensure correct placement. Both methods are effective, and their relative merits are debated. Bougie techniques give a better "feel" of the stricture which may be an important safety factor. Weighted non-wire-guided dilators

Cotton and Williams' Practical Gastrointestinal Endoscopy: The Fundamentals, Eighth Edition.
Catharine M. Walsh, Ahmir Ahmad, Brian P. Saunders, Jonathan Cohen, Peter B. Cotton, and Christopher B. Williams.
© 2024 John Wiley & Sons Ltd. Published 2024 by John Wiley & Sons Ltd.
Companion website: www.wiley.com/go/cottonwilliams8e

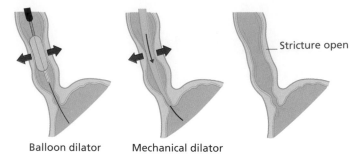

Fig 6.1 A balloon dilator exerts a radial force delivered simultaneously across the stricture, whereas a mechanical (push-type or bougie) dilator exerts a longitudinal and radial force, dilating proximal to distal on the stricture.

(such as tungsten-filled weighted rubber bougies) with blind insertion are seldom used now as safer dilators are available.

Certain strictures, particularly those due to irradiation or corrosive ingestion, are more difficult to dilate. Procedures may need to be repeated several times with a careful stepwise increase in dilator size (too rapid an increase can result in perforation) and endoscopic evaluation after dilation. As a general rule, no more than three dilators of progressively increasing size should be used during a single session.

Dilation is routinely performed in an outpatient setting. Anticoagulation medication should be discontinued. Routine antibiotic coverage is not recommended but dilation can provoke bacteremia, so antibiotic prophylaxis against endocarditis may be considered in patients with significant cardiac lesions (see Chapter 4).

Balloon dilation

Balloons are designed to be passed through the endoscope channel, often with a guidewire (Fig 6.2). They range from 3 to 8 cm in length and from 6 to 40 mm in diameter (some multidiameter with increasing pressures). Most strictures are short, but medium-length balloons (about 5 cm) are convenient to use, as they are less likely to "pop out" of the stricture than shorter ones. Lubrication makes insertion easier, either applied directly to the balloon with a silicone spray or by injecting 1–2 mL silicone oil down the endoscope channel followed by 10 mL air. The stricture is examined endoscopically, and its diameter is assessed. Tight strictures should be approached initially with small balloons, typically corresponding to the diameter of the stricture. The guidewire and soft tip of an appropriately sized balloon are passed gently through the stricture under direct vision. The balloons are fairly translucent, so that it is

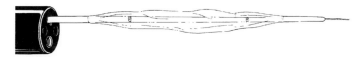

Fig 6.2 A deflated "through-the-scope" (TTS) balloon dilator and guidewire.

usually possible to observe the "waist" endoscopically during the procedure and to judge the effect. Balloons are distended with water (or contrast medium) to the pressure(s) recommended by the manufacturer conventionally for 1–2 minutes, although as little as 30 seconds may be sufficient.

The "through-the-scope" (TTS) balloon dilation technique has several advantages. It can be performed as part of the initial endoscopy and does not normally require fluoroscopic monitoring. The results should be obvious immediately, and the endoscope can be passed through the stricture to complete the endoscopic examination.

Bougie dilation

Dilation can be performed with graduated bougies that are passed over a guidewire. This ensures that the dilator will pass correctly through the stricture (and not into a diverticulum or necrotic tumor, or through the wall of a hiatus hernia). This security exists only if the position of the wire is checked frequently using fluoroscopy or a fixed external landmark. Fluoroscopic monitoring is essential when tight and complex strictures are being treated.

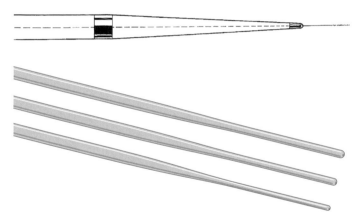

Fig 6.3 Tips of Savary-Gilliard (above) and American Endoscopy (below) dilators for use over a guidewire.

Savary-Gilliard bougies are popular. These are simple tapering plastic wands with radio-opaque markers (Fig 6.3). Variants of this design are available from other manufacturers. Diameters range from 3 to 20 mm.

The following steps should be performed when dilating:

1 *Place the guidewire* through the endoscope into the gastric antrum.

2 *Remove the scope and check the wire position* (Fig 6.4). This can be done fluoroscopically, or by checking the length of wire outside the patient. If the guidewire has distance markers, keep the 60 cm mark close to the patient's teeth.

3 *Choose a bougie* that will pass relatively easily through the stricture and slide it over the guidewire down close to the patient's mouth. Lubricate the tip of the bougie.

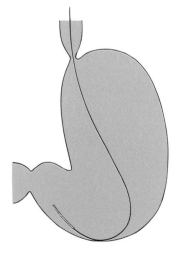

Fig 6.4 A dilator guidewire positioned in the gastric antrum.

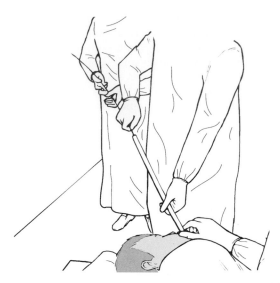

Fig 6.5 Advance the dilator with the left hand and the elbow extended to avoid sudden overinsertion. Keep traction on the wire with the right hand.

4 *Hold the bougie shaft in the left hand and push it in*, simultaneously applying countertraction on the guidewire with the right hand. Keep the left elbow extended so that the dilator cannot travel too far when resistance "gives" (Fig 6.5). This reduces the chance of advancing too rapidly.

5 *Increase the size of the bougies* progressively, checking the guidewire position repeatedly, but observe the rule of three; i.e. do not use more than three sizes above the size at which significant resistance is first felt.

6 *After dilation, check the effect endoscopically.* Take biopsy and cytology samples if necessary.

Refractory strictures

For some patients, an intensive dilation schedule and maximal gastroesophageal reflux therapy are not adequate to provide symptomatic relief. Several alternative endoscopic techniques have been used for such recalcitrant strictures.

• *Corticosteroid injection.* The injection of corticosteroids into a stricture is believed to reduce scar formation by preventing collagen deposition and enhancing local breakdown. Before stricture dilation, a standard sclerotherapy injection needle is used to deliver 0.5 mL triamcinolone acetonide (typically at 10–40 mg/mL) into each of the four quadrants of the narrowest area of the stricture. The evidence base for this practice is limited, but it appears to be beneficial in the treatment of anastomotic strictures and benign refractory esophageal strictures with evidence of inflammation.

• *Nonmetal stents.* Removable nonmetal stents have been introduced as an alternative for refractory strictures. Covered self-expanding plastic stents can be effective for benign strictures in the short term, but complications of stent migration and chest pain are common and limit overall clinical success. Biodegradable stents can also be effective in the short term (90 days) but also have a high rate of adverse events, and sequential stenting may be required to maintain clinical efficacy.

Post-dilation management

Patients should be kept nil by mouth and under observation for at least 1 hour after dilation. Any complaint of pain should be taken seriously. Chest films and a water-soluble contrast swallow should be performed if there is any suspicion of perforation (perforation is discussed in detail under "Esophageal cancer palliation" later in this chapter). A trial drink of water is given if progress has been satisfactory. The patient is then discharged with instructions to keep to a soft diet overnight, plus appropriate medications and a follow-up plan. Studies have shown that the use of proton pump inhibitors (PPIs) in patients with benign peptic strictures reduces the need for subsequent dilation when compared with H_2 antagonists and should therefore be added after the procedure. Dilation can be repeated within a few days in severe cases, and then subsequently every few weeks until swallowing has been fully restored.

Achalasia

Manometry provides the gold standard for the diagnosis of achalasia, but endoscopy is also essential to exclude submucosal or fundal malignancy. Achalasia can be treated with surgical or laparoscopic myotomy, per-oral endoscopic myotomy (POEM, discussed in Chapter 9), balloon dilation, or with injections of botulinum toxin. More recently, treatment using a hydrostatic dilation balloon has been described.

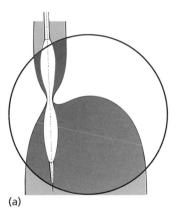

(a)

Balloon dilation

Patients with achalasia often have food residue in the esophagus. They should take only a clear liquid diet for several days before the procedure, and large-bore tube lavage may be needed beforehand.

Many different techniques and balloons have been used. The balloon position can be checked radiologically, or under direct vision with the endoscope alongside the balloon shaft (Fig 6.6), or even by a retroversion maneuver with the balloon fitted over the endoscope shaft. We prefer to place a guidewire endoscopically, identify the lower esophageal sphincter fluoroscopically, and then dilate with a balloon under fluoroscopic control.

Achalasia balloons are available with diameters of 30, 35, and 40 mm. It is wise to start with the smallest balloon, warning the patient that repeat treatments may be necessary if symptoms persist or recur quickly.

Inflation is maintained at the recommended pressure for up to 1 minute, and may be repeated. Observe the waist on the balloon fluoroscopically: inadequate expansion may indicate other pathology. Conversely, abrupt disappearance of the waist may suggest perforation.

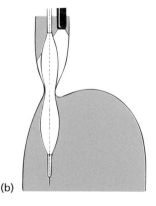

(b)

Fig 6.6 Achalasia dilating balloons (before full inflation) (a) checked fluoroscopically and (b) visualized endoscopically.

There is usually some blood on the balloon after the procedure. Close observation is mandatory for at least 4 hours. Chest radiographs and a water-soluble contrast swallow are done routinely in some units. Nothing should be given by mouth until the patient and the radiographs have been examined by the endoscopist personally. A trial drink of water is given under supervision and the uncomplicated patient can return to a normal diet on the next day.

Botulinum toxin

Treatment with botulinum toxin can be applied by direct free-hand endoscopic injection into the area of the lower esophageal sphincter, or using endoscopic ultrasound guidance. Reported results are good but short-lived, and the majority of patients require multiple procedures to maintain clinical efficacy. The value of this method may therefore be limited to individuals in whom other procedures are unacceptable or contraindicated.

Esophageal cancer palliation

Barium studies and endoscopy have complementary roles in assessing the site and nature of esophageal neoplasms. Endoscopic ultrasonography is the most accurate staging tool. Endoscopic management can help to improve swallowing in the majority of patients who are unsuitable for surgery because of intercurrent disease or tumor extent. However, endoscopists should be aware of their treatment limitations and should balance technological enthusiasm with full consideration of the patient's quality of life (and likely duration of survival). Achieving a large lumen will not restore normal swallowing. The goal should be to achieve adequate swallowing at the lowest risk and inconvenience to the patient.

Palliative techniques

Several methods can be used to palliate malignant dysphagia. The abrupt onset of severe dysphagia may be due to the impaction of a food bolus, which can be removed endoscopically by standard techniques. Malignant strictures can be dilated using wire-guided balloons or bougies, taking great care not to split the tumor by being overambitious. The bulk of an exophytic tumor can be reduced by various ablation techniques. Monopolar diathermy is readily available, but it is difficult to control the depth of injury, and charring occurs quickly. Local injection of a toxic agent such as absolute alcohol is also effective, if somewhat unpredictable. Laser ablation (using the Nd:YAG laser) was popular in previous years, largely because a "no-touch" technique seemed esthetically preferable, but the equipment is expensive, and similar results can be achieved using argon plasma coagulation (APC), which is simpler and cheaper. It also has the advantage that the energy can be applied tangentially.

Ablative techniques are most useful in short exophytic lesions, and for recurrences after surgery or stenting. All of the methods are somewhat hazardous (with a perforation rate of up to 5%) and are rarely effective for more than a few weeks. As a result, there is an increasing tendency to place stents as a primary measure. Chemotherapy, radiotherapy, and photodynamic therapy are also used.

Esophageal stenting

There are good indications for using esophageal stents, but insertion can be very challenging, and is not to be undertaken lightly by the endoscopist or patient. The best candidates are mid-esophageal tumors in patients with a prognosis limited to weeks or months, and in those with tracheoesophageal fistulae. Stents cannot be used when the tumor extends to within 2 cm of the cricopharyngeus. They may also function less well in lesions at the cardia because of the angulation, and reflux may be a problem. Newer stents with an anti-reflux mechanism may theoretically reduce this complication.

Great care must be taken when dysphagia is caused by very large tumors, as stent placement may compromise the airway. Prior bronchoscopy is appropriate in such cases, and trial inflation of a balloon may indicate which diameter is tolerable.

Stent variety

Traditional plastic stents with fixed diameters have largely been replaced by self-expandable metal or plastic stents (SEMS and SEPS, respectively), as they are easier and less hazardous to insert. Many types of **SEMS** are now available. They vary according to the type, diameter, and weave of the wires (which determine their expansile strength), their shapes and sizes, and the presence or absence of a covering membrane (Fig 6.7). This membrane is helpful in patients with fistulae, and reduces tumor ingrowth, but some mesh must be left exposed to prevent migration. Stents for use in the esophagus have luminal diameters of 15–24 mm, and lengths of 6–15 cm. They are compressed into delivery systems of 6–11 mm. Most expand gradually over a few days and become fully incorporated in the esophageal wall so that they cannot be removed. Less powerful stents—although easy to place and well tolerated—may not expand sufficiently to relieve the patient's symptoms, even with balloon dilation.

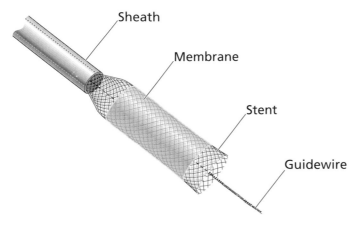

Fig 6.7 Covered metal mesh stent.

Newer **SEPS** are similar to SEMS in concept. The main advantage over metal stents is the ability to be repositioned or removed. Disadvantages include a larger, more difficult delivery system and higher migration rate. Currently, SEPS are indicated for benign esophageal diseases.

Stent insertion

Before insertion the patient should be fully informed about the aims of the procedure, the potential serious risks, and the (few) alternatives. The lesion is assessed carefully by radiology and endoscopy, and bougie dilation is performed, if necessary (to about 12 mm), to allow passage of the endoscope if possible. The upper and lower margins of the tumor are marked by endoscopic injection of contrast medium using a sclerotherapy needle, alternatively by taped external paperclip markers, or by endoscopic placement of metallic clips. A guidewire is placed, and its position checked by fluoroscopy.

The stent system is then introduced over the guidewire and the stent is released by gradual withdrawal of the sleeve. Correct positioning of the stent is judged fluoroscopically (using the contrast medium marks), and then by repeat endoscopy. Often the gastroscope is placed alongside the wire above the delivery system to monitor the deployment endoscopically.

Post-stent management

Patients are usually kept in the hospital overnight under observation because of the immediate risk of perforation and bleeding, and for necessary pain control. Clear fluids can be given after 4 hours if there have been no adverse developments.

Patients must understand the limitations of the stent, and the need to maintain a soft diet with plenty of fluids during and after meals. Written instructions should be provided, and relatives counseled. Overambitious eating or inadequate chewing may result in obstruction. If food impaction occurs, the bolus can usually be removed or fragmented endoscopically using snares, biopsy forceps, or balloons.

Stent dysfunction due to tumor overgrowth can be managed by endoscopic ablation or placement of another stent inside the first. SEPS offer the option of removal. Gastroesophageal reflux can be a problem with stents crossing the cardia. Patients may need to sleep propped up, and to use acid-reducing medications. Occasionally, a good result from chemotherapy or radiotherapy may make it possible to remove a stent. For the same reason, stents (especially the covered variety) may migrate spontaneously. Recovering stents from the stomach can be challenging.

Esophageal perforation

The endoscopic treatment of esophageal strictures is relatively safe in most cases using optimal techniques. Perforations do occur, however, especially with complex and malignant strictures approached by inexperienced or overconfident endoscopists. The rate is approximately 0.1% in benign esophageal strictures, 1% in achalasia dilation, and 5–10% in treatment of malignant lesions.

The risk is minimized by taking the process step by step—gradually and deliberately. Never try to dilate to the largest balloon or bougie simply because it is available. Additionally, using carbon dioxide for insufflation is especially important for endoscopic procedures with increased risk of perforation.

Early suspicion and recognition of perforation is the key to successful management, and no complaint should be ignored. The problem is usually obvious clinically; the patient is distressed and in pain. Signs of subcutaneous emphysema may develop within a few hours. Radiographic studies should be performed. Surgical consultation is mandatory when perforation is seriously suspected or confirmed. Many confined perforations have been managed conservatively, with nil oral intake, intravenous (IV) fluids, and broad-spectrum antibiotics—with or without placement of a nasogastric tube across the perforation.

Primary endoscopic closure of esophageal perforations should be pursued when feasible using through-the-scope clips or over-the-scope clips for perforations ≤2 cm and endoscopic suturing for larger perforations. Placement of a fully covered SEMS can be considered in cases where primary closure is not possible. Endoscopic vacuum therapy is a more recent technique to address large or persistent perforations whereby a vacuum system is applied through a nasogastric tube connected to a polyurethane sponge that is cut to size and inserted directly into the defect.

The choice between surgical and conservative management (and the timing of surgical intervention if conservative management appears to be failing) is often difficult; review of the literature shows varied and strong opinions. Conservative management is more likely to be appropriate when the perforation is in the neck; because the mediastinum is not contaminated, local surgical drainage can be performed simply when necessary. Perforation through a tumor can be treated immediately with a covered stent if the lumen can be found and if surgical cure is not possible.

For upper gastrointestinal tract perforations, a water-soluble upper gastrointestinal series should be considered to confirm the absence of continuing leakage at the perforation site before initiating a clear liquid diet.

Gastric and duodenal stenoses

Functionally significant stenoses may occur in the stomach or duodenum as a result of disease (tumors and ulcers) and following surgical intervention (e.g. hiatus hernia repair, gastroenterostomy, pyloroplasty, and gastroplasty). Balloon dilation of stenosed surgical stomas is usually effective (except in the case of banded gastroplasty with a rigid silicone ring). Pyloroduodenal stenosis caused by ulceration can be relieved by balloon dilation, but recurrence is common. Expandable stents are being used with remarkably good effect in patients with malignant stenosis of the stomach and duodenum. An emerging technique involves the use of short dumbbell-shaped lumen-apposing metal stents (LAMS) to create an anastomosis between the stomach and a loop of jejunum identified and accessed via endoscopic ultrasound.

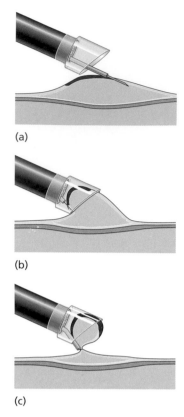

(a)

(b)

(c)

Fig 6.8 Endoscopic mucosal resection technique: (a) inject a saline cushion below the lesion; (b) suck the lesion into the transparent cap; and (c) snare and resect the lesion.

Gastric and duodenal polyps and tumors

Endoscopic polypectomy is frequently used in the colon, and many of the techniques (see Chapter 8) can be applied in the stomach and duodenum. Polyps are much less common in the stomach and duodenum than in the colon, and are rare in the esophagus. Many of these polyps are sessile, and some are largely submucosal, making endoscopic treatment more difficult and hazardous. The possibility of a transmural lesion should be considered, and endoscopic ultrasonography may be helpful in making a treatment decision; surgical (or laparoscopic) resection may be safer. Injecting the base of sessile gastric and duodenal polyps with epinephrine (adrenaline; 1:10,000) may make removal easier, and may reduce the risk of bleeding. Some endoscopists use detachable loops for the same purpose.

Endoscopic mucosal resection (EMR), originally developed in Japan, is used for en bloc removal of sessile or flat lesions up to 2 cm in diameter (or piecemeal if larger) confined to the superficial layers (mucosa and submucosa) of the gastrointestinal tract. In cap-assisted EMR, the lesion is raised up by injecting a cushion of saline/epinephrine, and then sucked into a special transparent plastic cap attached to the tip of the endoscope. The lesion is then resected with a snare loop incorporated in the cap (Fig 6.8). Other simpler methods of EMR are widely used, from the use of submucosal injection for lift prior to snare resection, which is employed frequently for large colon polyp resection, to the use of snare resection following band ligation of mucosal lesions, the so-called "band-EMR" or "ligation-assisted EMR" technique.

Snare diathermy techniques can also be used to obtain large biopsy specimens when the gastric mucosa appears thickened, and when standard biopsy techniques have failed to provide a diagnosis.

Gastric polypectomy, EMR, and snare loop biopsy techniques can cause bleeding and perforation. They also leave an ulcer; it is wise to prescribe acid-suppressant medication for a few weeks.

Foreign bodies

Foreign bodies are mainly a problem in children, elderly patients with poor teeth, those with psychiatric illness, and abusers of drugs or alcohol. The problem is obvious if the patient suddenly cannot swallow, and especially if a missing object is visible on a radiograph. However, many instances are less straightforward. Patients may not know that they have swallowed a foreign object. Some common items (e.g. bones and drink-can tags) are not radiopaque. It is therefore necessary to maintain a high index of suspicion.

Chest and abdominal radiographs (anterior-posterior and lateral views) are appropriate, as they may identify radiopaque objects or signs of esophageal perforation such as mediastinal or subcutaneous air. A water-soluble contrast swallow examination is helpful in some patients, but it is not necessary, and is potentially hazardous if dysphagia is complete.

Many foreign bodies pass spontaneously, but active treatment should be initiated within hours in some circumstances. Multiple magnets or a magnet and another metallic foreign body should be removed urgently (within 24 hours) due to the risk of pressure necrosis.

Emergency treatment (preferably within 2 hours of presentation, but at the latest within 6 hours) is required for:
• patients who cannot swallow saliva
• sharp-pointed objects in the esophagus
• button batteries in the esophagus (which cause local pressure necrosis, corrosive damage from leakage, and generation of an electrical current leading to hydroxide ion formation and an alkaline caustic injury).

Because of the potential for such life-threatening injury from button batteries, administration of honey and/or sucralfate (1 g/10 mL suspension) can be considered within 12 hours of presentation but should not delay endoscopy (dose: 10 mL) every 10 minutes with a maximum of six doses of honey and three doses of sucralfate). Following endoscopic removal, if signs of perforation are absent, acetic acid irrigation can be considered to neutralize accumulated tissue hydroxide with 50–150 mL 0.25% sterile acetic acid.

Foreign body retrieval

Objects impacted at or above the cricopharyngeal area are usually best removed by surgeons with rigid instruments. Flexible endoscopy now takes precedence in most (but not all) other situations. The use of an overtube increases the therapeutic options (Fig 6.9). Endoscopy can usually be accomplished with conscious sedation, but general anesthesia should be considered in children and uncooperative adults, and when there is concern about the airway being compromised.

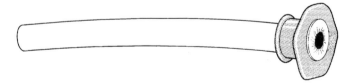

Fig 6.9 An overtube with biteguard.

Food impaction

If the patient is unable to tolerate their secretions, endoscopy should be performed emergently (ideally <2 hours from presentation), otherwise removal may be delayed up to 24 hours. An IV injection of glucagon (0.5–1 mg) has been used with equivocal results to release a food impaction by relaxing the esophagus, and such attempts at medical treatment should not delay endoscopy. The use of meat tenderizer is discouraged, as severe pulmonary complications have resulted. Meat can be removed as a single piece endoscopically, using a polypectomy snare, tri-prong grasper, or retrieval basket or net. Another approach is to use strong suction on the end of an overtube or a transparent cap taken from a banding device or purchased separately. Take care not to lose the bolus near the larynx. Food that has been impacted for several hours can usually be broken up (e.g. with a snare) and removed piecemeal, or the pieces pushed into the stomach. This must be done gently and very carefully, especially if there is any question of a bone being present. An overtube may be considered to minimize trauma with repeated esophageal intubations. At the time of endoscopy, biopsies should be taken from the proximal, mid, and distal esophagus to assess for underlying pathology, such as eosinophilic esophagitis, that would benefit from additional treatment and predispose to recurrence.

Most patients with impacted food have some esophageal narrowing (due to eosinophilic esophagitis, a benign reflux stricture or Schatzki ring). The endoscopist's task is not complete until this has been checked and treated. Sometimes it is possible to maneuver a small endoscope past the food bolus and to use the tip to dilate the distal stricture; the food can then be pushed through the narrowed area. Dilation can usually be performed at the time of food extraction, but it should be delayed if there is substantial edema or ulceration, or if there is suspicion for eosinophilic esophagitis, as biopsies should be obtained and reviewed, and appropriate treatment instituted.

Gastric bezoars

Gastric bezoars are aggregations of fibrous animal or vegetable material. They are usually found in association with delayed gastric emptying (e.g. postoperative stenosis or dysfunction). Most masses can be fragmented with biopsy forceps or a polypectomy snare, but more distal bolus obstruction may result if fragmentation is inadequate. Various enzyme preparations (e.g. cellulase) have been recommended to facilitate disruption, but these are rarely necessary or effective. Large gastric bezoars are best disrupted and removed by inserting a large-bore lavage tube and instilling and removing 2–3 L of tap water with a large syringe. Other techniques have included infusion of a carbonated drink, or mechanical or electrohydraulic or extracorporeal lithotripsy. The cause of gastric emptying dysfunction should be evaluated and treated.

Swallowed objects

The range of swallowed objects is amazing. Foreign bodies trapped in the esophagus should always be removed. Sharp objects (such as open safety pins) are best withdrawn into the tip of an overtube (Fig 6.10) or a latex hood (Fig 6.11). Rarely, it may be safer to use a rigid esophagoscope.

Most objects that reach the stomach will pass spontaneously, but there are exceptions that demand early intervention:
• sharp and pointed objects have a 15–35% chance of causing perforation (usually at the ileocecal valve), and should be extracted urgently (within 24 hours) while still in the stomach or proximal duodenum

Fig 6.10 Remove sharp foreign bodies with a protecting overtube.

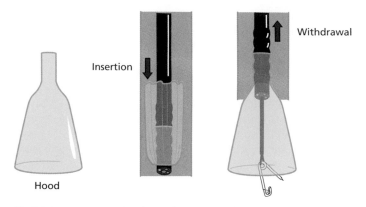

Fig 6.11 Latex hood for removal of small sharp objects.

• due to the risk of pressure necrosis, magnets should be removed urgently (within 24 hours)
• objects >2–2.5 cm diameter and longer than 5–6 cm are unlikely to pass the pylorus and duodenal curve spontaneously and should be removed urgently (within 24 hours).

Button batteries usually pass spontaneously when they have reached the stomach; a purgative should be given to accelerate the process. Gastric button batteries should be removed endoscopically if the patient is symptomatic, or the batteries have not passed into the small bowel within 7–14 days of ingestion. Those that do not pass into the stomach and remain in the esophagus should be removed emergently, as contact with the esophageal wall can quickly lead to liquefaction necrosis and perforation.

Foreign bodies rarely pass out of the stomach in children who have had pyloromyotomies.

Endoscopists should resist the temptation to attempt removal of illegal drugs (most often cocaine and heroin) packed in condoms or balloons, as rupture can lead to a massive overdose. Asymptomatic patients can be managed expectantly until the packets pass, with inpatient clinical observation, whole bowel irrigation, and radiographic follow-up. Use of polyethylene glycol lavage solutions are safe and likely accelerate the rate of clearance. For individuals with obstruction, perforation, or narcotic toxicity without an antidote (e.g. cocaine), immediate surgical evaluation and removal are the safest option.

Golden rules for foreign body removal:
• be sure that your retrieval procedure is really necessary
• think before you start, and rehearse outside the patient
• do not make the situation worse
• do not be slow to get surgical or anesthetic assistance
• protect the esophagus, pharynx, and bronchial tree during withdrawal (with an overtube or endotracheal anesthesia)
• remove sharp objects with the point trailing and use a protective device (e.g. latex rubber hood, overtube, transparent cap) to prevent mucosal injury during extraction (Table 6.1).

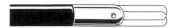

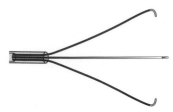

Fig 6.12 Foreign body grasping (extraction) forceps.

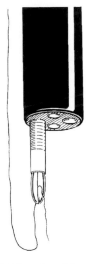

Fig 6.13 A triprong grasping device.

Fig 6.14 Take a thread down with the forceps to pass through any object with a hole in it, such as a ring or key.

Retrieval devices

The endoscopist should have several specialized tools available, in addition to the overtube (Table 6.1). There are forceps with claws or flat blades designed to grasp coins (Fig 6.12); a tri-prong extractor is useful for meat (Fig 6.13). Many objects can be grasped with a polypectomy snare or stone-retrieval basket. Others can be collected in a retrieval net. A protector hood can be placed at the tip of the endoscope to protect the esophageal and pharyngeal wall from sharp edges of the foreign body during extraction (Fig 6.11). Any object with a hole (such as a key or ring) can be removed by passing a thread through the hole. The endoscope is passed into the stomach with biopsy forceps or a snare closed within its tip, grasping a thread, which passes down the outside of the instrument (Fig 6.14). The forceps are advanced, and the thread passed through the object, dropped, and retrieved from the other side.

Prior to endoscopy, it can be useful to practice grasping a similarly sized object to determine the most appropriate retrieval device.

Table 6.1 Retrieval devices

Object type	Possible retrieval devices
Blunt object	Grasping forceps, grasping device, polypectomy snare, retrieval basket or net
Sharp-pointed object	Grasping forceps, polypectomy snare, retrieval basket or net Protection device: latex rubber hood, overtube, transparent cap
Long object	Polypectomy snare, retrieval basket
Food bolus	Grasping forceps, grasping device, polypectomy snare, retrieval basket or net Protection device: overtube for repeated esophageal intubations

Acute bleeding

Acute upper gastrointestinal bleeding (hematemesis and/or melena) is a common medical problem for which endoscopy has become the primary diagnostic and therapeutic technique. Emergency endoscopy is a challenging task. There is considerable potential for benefit, but also for risk. These techniques require experience, nerve, and judgment. Safety considerations are paramount. The endoscopist should be well trained, working with familiar equipment and expert nurses. Unstable patients should be under supervision in an intensive care environment. Sedation should be given cautiously, and precautions taken to avoid pulmonary aspiration. Patients with severe bleeding are often best examined under general anesthesia, with the airway protected by a cuffed endotracheal tube.

Many different endoscopic techniques have been developed. These include injection with absolute ethanol or saline/epinephrine or sclerosant (e.g. sodium tetradecyl sulfate) or glue, banding, thermal probes (heater probe, bipolar, or monopolar electrocoagulation, APC, and lasers), clipping and hemostatic powder spray, and endoscopic suturing. Many trials have compared different techniques. The appropriate hemostasis techniques and the correct application of each (including power settings) is well documented in the literature. For certain lesions, such as ulcers with actively bleeding visible vessels or nonbleeding visible vessels, dual modality treatment has been shown to be superior to injection monotherapy, and this usually takes the form of injection plus direct contact thermal therapy or injection plus clip application. Laser photocoagulation initially became popular because it was assumed that it was safer not to touch the lesion. It has become clear, however, that direct pressure with some probes (and injection treatment) provides an important tamponade and "coaptation" effect (Fig 6.20) and increases the size of vessel that can be treated. Certain other newer therapies have been introduced for refractory acute bleeding that include use of hemostatic sprays, over-the-scope large clips, and endoscopic suturing. It is important to review principles of electrocautery and familiarize oneself with the electrosurgical unit used in one's endoscopy unit and the generator settings used for different purposes.

The *timing* of endoscopy is important. Examination can be delayed to a convenient time (e.g. the next morning) in patients who appear to be stable, but the endoscopic team must be prepared to go into action within hours (after immediate resuscitation) in certain circumstances and in other lower-risk situations within 24 hours of presentation. Several validated systems exist to risk stratify patients for endoscopy, including the Rockall Score and the Glasgow-Blatchford Score (Tables 6.2 and 6.3).

Indications for emergency endoscopy include:
- continued active bleeding requiring intervention
- suspicion of variceal bleeding
- presence of an aortic graft
- severe rectal bleeding with inconclusive colonic studies
- elderly patients with cardiovascular compromise on presentation.

Table 6.2 Rockall Score

	0	1	2	3
Age (years)	<60	60–79	>79	–
Degree of shock	Systolic BP >100 mmHg Heart rate <100/min	Systolic BP >100 mmHg Heart rate >100/min	Systolic BP <100 mmHg Heart rate >100/min	–
Comorbidities	None	–	Heart failure Ischemic heart disease	Renal/liver failure Disseminated cancer
Endoscopic diagnosis	Mallory-Weiss tear No lesion	All other diagnosis	Upper GI malignancy	–
Stigmata of bleeding	None or dark spot only	–	Visible/spurting vessel, blood, clot	–

Table 6.3 Glasgow-Blatchford Score

(a) Blood urea (mmol/L)	Score	(c) Systolic BP (mmHg)	Score
6.5 – 7.9	2	100 – 109	1
8.0 – 9.9	3	90 – 99	2
10.0 – 24.9	4	<90	3
≥25	6	**(d) Other markers**	
(b1) Hemoglobin for men (g/dL)		Pulse ≥100 beats/min	1
12.0 – 12.9	1	Presentation with melena	1
10.0 – 11.9	3	Presentation with syncope	2
<10.0	6	Hepatic disease*	2
(b2) Hemoglobin for women (g/dL)		Cardiac failure*	2
10.0 – 11.9	1		
<10.0	6		

*Hepatic disease and cardiac failure were not defined in the original score. However, a more recent study defined hepatic disease as a known history, or clinical and laboratory evidence, of chronic or acute liver disease, and cardiac failure as known history, or clinical and echocardiographic evidence, of cardiac failure.

Gastric lavage

Blood clots may obscure the view in the stomach and duodenum. Standard gastric lavage is rarely effective, even when performed personally with a large-bore tube. Endoscopes with a large channel (or two channels) allow better flushing and suction. An alternative approach is to start the procedure with an overtube over the endoscope (Fig 6.15). If blood is encountered, the endoscope can be removed, and blood clots sucked directly through the overtube; lavage can then be performed. In such cases, serious consideration must be given to seeking anesthesia support for intubation to protect the airway from aspiration.

A diagnosis can usually be made even if the stomach cannot be emptied completely. Lesions are rare on the greater curvature, where the blood pools in the standard left lateral position. Changing the patient's position somewhat should improve the survey but turning completely on the right side is hazardous unless the airway is protected.

An alternative to lavage may be the use of pharmacologic agents, such as erythromycin, to accelerate gastric emptying. Studies have shown that a single dose of IV erythromycin (250 mg) 20–90 minutes prior to endoscopy can significantly improve visibility, reducing the need for second-look endoscopy and length of hospitalization.

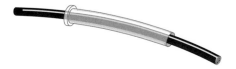

Fig 6.15 Overtube with endoscope.

Bleeding lesions

Lesions that cause acute bleeding are well known. Endoscopy has highlighted the fact that many patients are found to have more than one mucosal lesion (e.g. esophageal varices and acute gastric erosions). Thus, a complete examination of the esophagus, stomach, and duodenum should be performed in every bleeding patient, no matter what is seen en route. A lesion should be incriminated as the bleeding source only if it is actively bleeding at the time of endoscopy, or shows characteristic stigmata, for example, an ulcer with an adherent clot or a visible vessel. If the patient has presented with hematemesis, and complete upper endoscopy shows only a single lesion (even without any of these features), it is likely to be the bleeding source. This is not necessarily the case if the presentation has been with melena, or if the examination takes place more than 48 hours after bleeding, since acute lesions such as mucosal tears and erosions may already have healed. Likewise, varices cannot be incriminated definitely unless they are bleeding or show specific stigmata.

Variceal treatments

Endoscopic treatment of esophageal (and gastric) varices can be helpful in patients who are bleeding, or who have recently bled. Prophylactic endoscopic treatment for primary prevention (i.e. to prevent the first variceal bleed) remains controversial. Intervention in the presence of active bleeding is challenging, but a very high rate of immediate bleeding control is possible. Patients are often very sick, and the views may be poor. It may be helpful to tilt the patient slightly head up, or to apply traction on a gastric balloon to reduce the flow of blood as a temporary measure. Successful management necessitates aggressive hemodynamic resuscitation of the patient, often with anticoagulation and transfusion, along with airway protection to prevent aspiration. Actively or recently bleeding esophageal varices are most commonly managed endoscopically with the application of band ligation to suction up and obliterate the varices. Elimination of varices usually involves a series of treatments. The use of injection sclerotherapy for esophageal varices with agents such as ethanolamine has largely been discontinued due to higher rates of adverse events, including ulceration and strictures. In many countries, the use of cyanoacrylate glue injection has proven effective for use in esophageal and especially gastric varices, for which band ligation alone leads to very high rates of rebleeding.

Other endoscopic tools have been applied in the control of variceal bleeding, including the use of hemostatic spray to achieve temporary control when other methods are not possible or working, tamponade using a covered self-expanding metal stent, or detachable snares/loop or over-the-scope large clips. An important salvage procedure, particularly for gastric varices, is the use of transjugular intrahepatic portosystemic shunt (TIPS) by interventional radiology, embolization of varices with coils and/or glue via interventional radiology, or endoscopic ultrasound needle injection. Occasionally, in unstable patients in whom standard endoscopic methods cannot control the bleeding, bleeding may be temporarily controlled by tamponade using a Sengstaken-Blakemore tube placed down the esophagus, inflated in the stomach, and pulled up to the gastroesophageal junction under traction. There is a high rate of adverse events associated with this rarely used technique, which is employed only as a bridge to stabilize the patient for a more definitive treatment like a TIPS.

All patients with cirrhosis presenting with acute upper GI bleeding need to be given prophylactic antibiotics, regardless of the ultimate identified bleeding source (variceal or nonvariceal) or treatment modality used.

Variceal banding

Banding is now considered the procedure of choice for esophageal varices because it causes fewer ulcers and strictures than sclerotherapy and has a proven mortality benefit. Commercially available devices consist of a friction-fit sleeve for the endoscope tip, an inner cylinder preloaded with elastic bands, and a trip wire that passes up the endoscope channel (Fig 6.16). The varix is sucked into the sleeve, and the band is released by pulling on the wire. Multiple bands are applied in an upward spiral fashion every 1–2 cm.

Banding can also be applied to gastric varices and to small ulcers (e.g. Dieulafoy lesions). Disadvantages to the band ligator include obscured visibility by blood during active bleeding, and poor maneuverability.

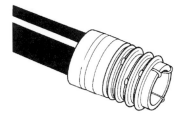

Fig 6.16 An esophageal banding device.

Injection sclerotherapy and glue injection

Injection sclerotherapy is not recommended as the standard of care in acute esophageal variceal hemorrhage; however, endoscopic cyanoacrylate glue injection is the treatment of choice for acute bleeding from gastric varices. Sclerotherapy using chemical agents such as sodium tetradecyl sulfate or ethanolamine is still used in small infants (generally less than 8–10 kg) where banding is not possible.

Many adjuvant devices have been described, including overtubes with a lateral window and the use of balloons, either in the stomach to compress distal varices or on the scope itself to permit tamponade if bleeding occurs. However, most experts use a simple "free-hand" method, with a standard large-channel endoscope and a flexible, retractable needle (Fig 6.17). Injections are given directly into the varices, starting close to the cardia (and below any bleeding site) and working spirally upward for about 5 cm. Each injection consists of 1–2 mL of sclerosant, to a total of 20–40 mL (10–15 mL in children, depending on size) per session.

Precise placement of the needle within the varix (as guided by co-injection of a dye such as methylene blue or by simultaneous manometric or radiographic techniques) may improve the results and reduce the risk of adverse events. However, some experts believe that paravariceal injections are also effective, and it is often difficult to tell which has been achieved. If bleeding occurs on removal of the needle, it is usually helpful to tamponade the

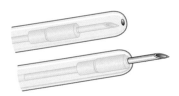

Fig 6.17 A retractable sclerotherapy needle.

area simply by passing the endoscope into the stomach. The gastroesophageal junction can be compressed directly if the endoscope is retroflexed.

For glue injection, the needle (21–23 gauge) is flushed with distilled water initially (normal saline is not used, as it delays solidification of glue). The glue is injected directly into the gastric varix adjacent to the bleeding site. Each injection consists of 0.5–1 mL of pure glue followed immediately by 1 mL of distilled water to flush the channel while the needle is still in the varix. Further injections of glue, in 0.5–1 mL aliquots, are given until complete hemostasis is achieved, and the varix is solidified. Any tributaries entering the main varix should also be injected. Acetone should be kept ready to clean the endoscope tip or channel in case the glue spills.

Chemical sclerosants have now largely been replaced by endoscopic injection of a tissue adhesive such as cyanoacrylate glue. These polymers solidify almost immediately on contact with aqueous material. The endoscopist and nurse must use them carefully to provide an effective injection without gluing up the endoscope. Results are excellent, especially in gastric varices (which do not respond well to standard sclerotherapy), where this technique is used routinely to treat acute bleeding.

Care after variceal treatments

The risks of variceal treatment include all of the complications of emergency endoscopy (especially pulmonary aspiration).

Patients often have transient chest pain, odynophagia (pain on swallowing), and dysphagia. They should maintain a soft diet for a few days, avoid any medications that may irritate or cause bleeding, and take acid-suppressing agents. Ulcerations form at the site of band ligation when the bands fall off and these may also be a source of rebleeding, particularly in patients with significant coagulation abnormalities secondary to underlying liver disease. Variceal treatment should be repeated in 1–2 weeks in the context of acute bleeding, but should be delayed for several weeks, when elective, to allow the lesions to heal. Delayed adverse events include esophageal stricturing, which is more common after sclerotherapy. Strictures can be dilated gingerly with standard methods.

Treatment of bleeding ulcers

Duodenal and gastric ulcers are still common causes of acute bleeding. About 80% will stop bleeding spontaneously. It is important, if possible, to predict those patients likely to rebleed and to select them for endoscopic treatment. We are guided by the size of the initial bleed, the overall status of the patient, and by the presence or absence of stigmata.

Ulcer stigmata

The following stigmata provide useful pointers when considering treatment options:
• *Active "spurters"* (Forrest 1a) continue to bleed (or rebleed soon) in 70–80% of cases.
• *Ulcers with an oozing bleed* (Forrest 1b) continue to bleed (or rebleed soon) in 50% of cases.

- *Ulcers with a nonbleeding "visible vessel"* (Forrest IIa) have about a 40–50% chance of rebleeding.
- *Ulcers with an "adherent clot"* (Forrest IIb) have about a 20–30% chance of rebleeding.
- *Ulcers with a flat spot in the ulcer base* (Forrest IIc) have about a 7–10% chance of rebleeding.
- *Clean ulcers generally do not rebleed* (Forrest III).

An important question is whether it is appropriate to wash clots off the base of an ulcer simply to check for these stigmata. Most endoscopists will do so in high-risk patients provided they are poised for treatment.

Treatment modalities

The endoscopic hemostatic methods currently recommended for bleeding due to ulcers are bipolar electrocoagulation, heater probe, and absolute ethanol injection. Through the scope clips and other mechanical closure devices, argon plasma coagulation and soft monopolar electrocoagulation are other modalities that may be efficacious when used alone or in combination. Hemostatic powder spray may also be a useful noncontact endoscopic option to temporize massive bleeding where it is not possible to perform thermal therapy or hemoclip placement. Large over-the-scope clips and endoscopic suturing methods have also been successfully applied to treat refractory nonvariceal bleeding lesions.

- *Injection treatment*. Absolute ethanol is applied with a sclerotherapy needle in 0.1–0.2 mL aliquots around the base of the of the bleeding site, up to a total of 1–2 mL to minimize tissue injury. Epinephrine in saline (1:10,000 to 1:100,000 dilution, 0.5–2 mL aliquots, up to 10 mL) can be used in combination with other hemostatic modalities but is not recommended to be used alone. At least some of the utility of this injection is a tamponade effect. It is well established that injection therapy alone is inferior to thermal or mechanical hemostasis methods for treatment of ulcer bleeding, so injection is usually used in combination with one of these other modalities.
- The *heater probe* (Fig 6.18) provides a constant temperature of 250°C. First tamponade, then apply several pulses of 30 J.
- The *bipolar (or multipolar) probe* (Fig 6.19) provides bipolar electrocoagulation, which is assumed to be safer than monopolar diathermy (which produces an unpredictable depth of damage). Use the larger 10 French gauge probe at 30–40 W for 10 seconds.
- Newer *monopolar hemostatic forceps with soft coagulation* work at a lower voltage than traditional monopolar probes resulting in less tissue damage. The closed tip of the forceps is firmly applied to the bleeding site using soft coagulation mode at settings of 50–80 W with 1- to 2-second applications, or the forceps can be used to grasp the bleeding point. Such brief precise soft coagulation of tissue at high wattage sears the vessel itself but delivers less deep thermal injury than monopolar coagulation.

These treatment devices share some common principles. All can be applied tangentially, but (apart from injection) are better used face-on if possible. When the vessel is actively bleeding, direct

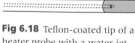

Fig 6.18 Teflon-coated tip of a heater probe with a water-jet opening.

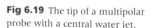

Fig 6.19 The tip of a multipolar probe with a central water jet.

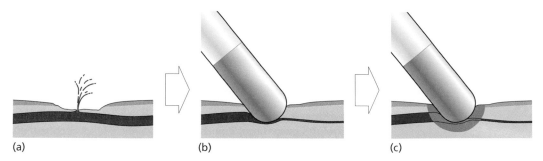

Fig 6.20 (a) When an ulcer is actively bleeding, (b) probe pressure stops the blood flow and coapts the vessel wall (c) with subsequent thermal coagulation.

probe pressure on the vessel or feeding vessel (i.e. coaptive coagulation) will reduce the flow and increase the effectiveness of treatment (Fig 6.20). The bipolar and heater probes incorporate a flushing water jet, which helps to prevent sticking.

• ***Combination therapy*** involves injection of epinephrine followed by application of thermal coaptive coagulation. Some prefer to inject epinephrine after clip application to avoid local swelling that can make placement more difficult or to treat residual bleeding after clip application.

• ***Clipping*** (Fig 6.21). Metal clips can be applied endoscopically and are particularly useful for small bleeding ulcers (e.g. Dieulafoy lesions), Mallory-Weiss tears, and large visible vessels.

• ***Over-the-scope clips*** may be useful in recurrent ulcer bleeding after successful endoscopic hemostasis. A cap device with a single clip is placed over the ulcer to encircle it, the lesion is sucked into the cap, and the clip is released.

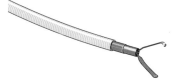

Fig 6.21 Hemostatic clip.

• To administer ***hemostatic powder spray***, place the tip of the delivery catheter 1 to 2 cm from the bleeding site and apply the powder in short 1- to 2-second bursts until the bleeding site is covered and bleeding stops. This is best used as a temporizing measure when conventional endoscopic therapies are not available or fail and is a particularly useful noncontact endoscopic option for massive or diffuse bleeding, poor visualization, or salvage therapy. It should be followed by a second-look endoscopy and/or a definitive hemostatic modality as the powder sloughs off the mucosa within 24 hours after application and the powder does not induce tissue healing.

• ***Argon plasma coagulation*** is a noncontact mode of thermal hemostasis in which a high voltage is delivered to inert argon gas at the tip of a probe to make a plasma. The plasma seeks a ground and the tissue in front of or to the side of the tip of the probe is desiccated and coagulated. While it has only seen limited use for bleeding peptic ulcers due to lack of direct tamponade on the vessel, this modality has been used widely for bleeding due to angioectasias.

• ***Full-thickness endoscopic sutures*** are now available and have been reported in use to perform hemostasis of difficult acute nonvariceal upper GI bleeding.

Many of these modalities may be used to treat other nonvariceal causes of upper and lower GI bleeding besides ulcers.

Know when to stop treatment!

Treatment attempts should not be protracted if major difficulties are encountered; the risks rise as time passes. There are some patients and lesions in which endoscopic intervention may be foolhardy, and surgery is more appropriate, for example, a large posterior wall duodenal ulcer that may involve the gastroduodenal artery. Angiographic treatment is useful in selected cases.

Follow-through after treatment

A single endoscopic treatment is not an all-or-nothing event. It is necessary to continue other medical measures, to maintain close monitoring, and to plan ahead for further intervention (pharmacological, endoscopic, radiological, or surgical) if bleeding continues or recurs. The job is not complete until the lesion is fully healed. IV, followed by oral, PPI post-endoscopic treatment and eradication of *Helicobacter pylori*, should reduce the risk of late rebleeding.

Treatment of bleeding vascular lesions

All of the endoscopic methods can be used to treat vascular malformations such as angiomas and telangiectasia. The risk of full-thickness damage and perforation is greater in organs with thinner walls (e.g. the esophagus and duodenum) than in the stomach. Lesions with a diameter of more than 1 cm should be approached with caution and treated from the periphery inward to avoid provoking hemorrhage. Bipolar and heater probes and APC provide the best control. Many endoscopists inject submucosal saline to provide a cushion prior to APC in thin-walled locations.

Complications of hemostasis

The most important hazards of endoscopic hemostasis are pulmonary aspiration and provocation of further bleeding. It is difficult to know how often endoscopy causes rebleeding that would not have occurred spontaneously, but major immediate bleeding is unusual and can usually be stopped. The risk of pulmonary aspiration is minimized by protecting the airway using pharyngeal suction and a head-down position, or a cuffed endotracheal tube. Perforation can be caused by any of the treatment methods if they are used too aggressively, especially in acute ulcers, which have little protecting fibrosis.

Enteral nutrition

There are several ways in which endoscopists can assist patients who need nutritional help. Temporary support can be provided by placement of a nasoenteric feeding tube. Long-term nutritional support requires the creation of a gastrostomy (or jejunostomy).

Feeding and decompression tubes

Tubes for short-term feeding (and gastric decompression) are normally placed blindly at the bedside but can also be passed under fluoroscopic guidance or after endoscopic placement of a guidewire.

Two direct endoscopic methods can be used when necessary, for example, to advance tubes through the pylorus or a surgical stoma. These are the *through-the-channel method* and the *along-the-scope method*.

Through-the-channel method

This is the simplest technique and entails advancing a 7–8 French gauge plastic tube through a large-channel endoscope, over a standard (400 cm long) 0.035-inch-diameter guidewire (Fig 6.22). The tube and guidewire are advanced through the pylorus under direct vision, and subsequent passage is checked by fluoroscopy. When the tip is in the correct position, the endoscope is withdrawn while further advancing the tube (and guidewire) through it. Finally, the guidewire is removed, and the tube is rerouted through the nose. Another method is to pass a guidewire through the biopsy channel into position in the small bowel. The endoscope is then removed, and a feeding tube is fed over the guidewire into position.

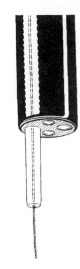

Fig 6.22 The feeding tube and guidewire are passed through a large-channel scope.

Alongside-the-scope method

This technique allows the placement of a tube larger than the endoscope channel. The feeding tube is stiffened with one or more guidewires. A short length of suture material is attached to the end of the tube and is grasped within the instrument channel with a snare (Fig 6.23). The endoscope is passed into the stomach and close to the pylorus. The snare and tube are then guided through the pylorus (or stoma) under direct vision. Once in position (checked by fluoroscopy), the thread is released, and the endoscope is removed. The proximal end of the tube is rerouted from the mouth to the nose. The final position is checked by fluoroscopy, withdrawing any excess loops in the stomach.

A variant of this method has proven useful. The feeding tube (again stiffened with one or more guidewires) is passed through the nose and into the stomach. The endoscope is passed through the mouth and is used to push the tip of the tube through the pylorus. The endoscope is then passed alongside the tube into the duodenum. The tube advances by the friction between the scope and the tube. The tube is held firmly at the nose, and the scope is withdrawn to the pylorus and then advanced again to push the tube deeper.

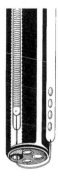

Fig 6.23 A tube is carried alongside the scope by a thread grasped with a snare or forceps.

Percutaneous endoscopic gastrostomy (PEG)

Nasoenteric feeding can be used for several weeks but is inconvenient and unstable, and it is probably often responsible for pulmonary aspiration and pneumonia. PEG is now a popular method for long-term feeding in patients who are unable to maintain adequate volitional intake and may permit the transfer of patients with chronic neurological disability from acute care hospitals to home or long-term care facilities. The PEG technique can be extended into a feeding jejunostomy by the use of appropriate tubes.

Studies comparing PEG with open or laparoscopic gastrostomy (performed by surgeons) and fluoroscopy-guided gastrostomy

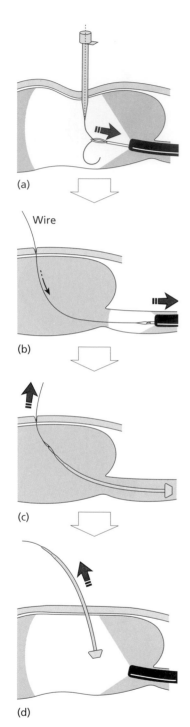

(a)

Wire

(b)

(c)

(d)

Fig 6.24 PEG insertion technique: (a) Grasp the wire; (b) pull the wire through the mouth; (c) pull the PEG tube down the esophagus; and (d) pull bumper to gastric wall.

(performed by interventional radiologists) have shown some advantages for the endoscopic method, but surgical or radiologic options should always be considered, especially in circumstances where the endoscopic approach may be more difficult or hazardous (e.g. after gastric surgery).

Antibiotics are usually given to reduce the risk of skin sepsis.

There are two main methods for PEG placement: the "pull" and the "push" methods.

The "pull" technique

This, the original method, is still the most commonly used.

1 *A standard endoscope is passed, and the gastric outlet is checked*.

2 *The patient is rotated onto the back, the stomach distended with air, and the room darkened* (this is particularly important when using videoscopes).

3 *The tip of the endoscope is directed toward the anterior wall* of the stomach.

4 *The assistant observes the abdominal wall for transillumination* and indents the site with a finger.

5 *The endoscopist checks the indentation site* to be sure it is in an appropriate part of the body of the stomach.

6 *The assistant marks this spot on the anterior abdominal wall*, applies disinfectant, and infiltrates local anesthetic into the skin, subcutaneous tissues, and fascia.

7 *A 5–10 mm skin incision is made* with a pointed blade, extending into the subcutaneous fat.

8 *The assistant inserts an 18 gauge needle catheter* (loaded onto a syringe half full of water) through the anterior abdominal wall, aspirating after initial penetration. Air should not bubble back until the needle is visible endoscopically (showing that it is in the stomach, not in another organ such as the colon).

9 *The endoscopist places a snare in front of the area of indentation and needle entry* and maintains gastric distension.

10 *A string is passed through the needle and is grasped with the snare* (the string has loops at both ends and must be at least 150 cm long) (Fig 6.24a).

11 *The endoscope and snare are withdrawn through the mouth* (Fig 6.24b) carrying the string, while ensuring that the external end of the string remains outside the abdominal wall.

12 *The PEG tube is attached to the string loop coming out of the mouth, then pulled down the esophagus (Fig 6.24c) and through the anterior abdominal wall* (Fig 6.24d). The tube should not be pulled tight, to avoid compression necrosis of the gastric wall. Leave about 1 cm of "play," as judged endoscopically.

13 *The tube is shortened and then anchored at the skin* with one of various disk devices.

Feeding can start on the day after the procedure (with a trial of water initially) if there are no adverse events. The patient and all relevant caregivers are given detailed instructions on tube care, and what to do if problems arise. After about 2 months the initial tube can usually be replaced with a flat feeding button.

The "push" technique

This follows steps 1 through 8 above, to the point where the needle catheter is in the stomach, with the endoscope poised in front of it. A long straight guidewire is then pushed through the needle and grasped endoscopically with a snare. The scope and snare are removed via the mouth, so that there is a long wire extending from the mouth through the stomach and through the abdominal wall. Keeping tension on both ends of the wire, a special PEG tube is then slid all the way over the wire. The tip of the tube is grasped as it exits the abdominal wall and pulled into place. An external bolster is attached.

Direct introducer technique

This is used in some countries, especially by radiologists. The feeding tube is pushed through the abdominal wall, rather than pulling it down from the mouth. The stomach is distended with air using a nasogastric tube under fluoroscopy. A needle catheter, trochar, and straight guidewire are passed through the abdominal wall into the stomach. A succession of dilators are passed over the wire, and eventually a PEG tube in a sleeve. The sleeve is removed, and the PEG withdrawn into position. This method eliminates contamination of the PEG tube by passage through the mouth, but it is difficult to choose the correct puncture position unless endoscopy is used. It is sometimes also difficult to push the trochar and catheter through the abdominal and stomach walls. A new variant of this technique (PEX-ACT) uses specialized needles and loops to create sutures anchoring the stomach wall to the abdominal wall before insertion of the large-bore PEG tube. Again, this requires internal visualization using an endoscope.

PEG problems and risks

PEG placement cannot be performed in patients with esophageal strictures that are too tight to permit the passage of an endoscope. Technical difficulties and risks are higher in patients who have previously undergone abdominal surgery, particularly with partial gastric resection, and in patients with gastric varices, marked ascites, or obesity.

Specific risks of PEG

There are three main types of risk.
- *Perforation/fistula.* Avoid injuring other organs (such as the colon) by making sure that good transillumination is achieved, and by using the bubble-back check. A small pneumoperitoneum is not uncommon, and is usually benign, but major and persisting leakage requires operative correction.
- *Local infection* can occur (even necrotizing fasciitis), particularly if the skin incision is too small or if the tube has been pulled too tight against the gastric wall (one of the most common errors). Pre-procedure antibiotics reduce this risk.
- *Tube dislodgement* can result in peritonitis and may require surgical repair. Dislodgement after 10–14 days usually leaves a track (for 12–24 hours) during which the tube can be replaced (with care).

Percutaneous endoscopic jejunostomy (PEJ)

Jejunal feeding is often recommended to reduce the risk of pulmonary aspiration, especially in patients with gastroesophageal reflux and gastroparesis. The jejunostomy tube may be inserted (under endoscopic guidance) through an established PEG tract or using special commercial kits at the time of the original PEG puncture (PEG-J). The technique for placing the tip of the tube in the jejunum is similar to the "alongside-the-scope" method for nasojejunal tubes described earlier. Placing a jejunostomy tube directly into the small bowel, by analogous transillumination/puncture techniques, has been done and obviates the need for surgery or interventional radiology but does carry higher risks compared with PEJ/PEG-J.

Nutritional support

The purpose of these endoscopic interventions is to provide safe and effective nutritional support. It is thus important to ensure that the patient and all involved caregivers are instructed appropriately about tube care and feeding regimens. They also need structured follow-up and support.

Further reading

Neoplasia

Ahmed O, Lee JH, Thompson CC, et al. AGA Clinical practice update on the optimal management of the malignant alimentary tract obstruction: Expert review. *Clin Gastroenterol Hepatol* 2021;19(9):1780–8.

ASGE Standards of Practice Committee, Evans JA, Early DS, et al. The role of endoscopy in the assessment and treatment of esophageal cancer. *Gastrointest Endosc* 2013;77(3):328–34.

ASGE Standards of Practice Committee, Evans JA, Chandrasekhara V, et al. The role of endoscopy in the management of premalignant and malignant conditions of the stomach. *Gastrointest Endosc* 2015;82(1):1–8.

ASGE Standards of Practice Committee, Jue TL, Storm AC, et al. ASGE guideline on the role of endoscopy in the management of benign and malignant gastroduodenal obstruction. *Gastrointest Endosc* 2021;93(2): 309–22.

ASGE Technology Committee, Varadarajulu S, Banerjee S, et al. Enteral stents. *Gastrointest Endosc* 2011;74(3):455–64.

Foreign bodies

ASGE Standards of Practice Committee, Ikenberry SO, Jue TL, et al. Management of ingested foreign bodies and food impactions. *Gastrointest Endosc* 2011;73(6):1085–91.

Birk M, Bauerfeind P, Deprez PH, et al. Removal of foreign bodies in the upper gastrointestinal tract in adults: European Society of Gastrointestinal Endoscopy (ESGE) Clinical Guideline. *Endoscopy* 2016;48(5):489–96.

Kramer RE, Lerner DG, Lin T, et al. Management of ingested foreign bodies in children: A clinical report of the NASPGHAN Endoscopy Committee. *J Pediatr Gastroenterol Nutr* 2015;60(4):562–74.

Mubarak A, Benninga MA, Broekaert I, et al. Diagnosis, management, and prevention of button battery ingestion in childhood: A European

Society for Paediatric Gastroenterology Hepatology and Nutrition Position Paper. *J Pediatr Gastroenterol Nutr* 2021;73(1):129–36.

Nutrition

ASGE Standards of Practice Committee, Jain R, Maple JT, et al. The role of endoscopy in enteral feeding. *Gastrointest Endosc* 2011;74(1):7–12.

DeLegge MH, Sabol DA. Provision for enteral and parenteral support. In: Bales CW, Ritchie CS, eds. *Handbook of Clinical Nutrition and Aging* (1st edition). Totowa, NJ: Humana Press, 2004:583–95.

Bleeding

ASGE Standards of Practice Committee, Gurudu SR, Bruining DH, et al. The role of endoscopy in the management of suspected small-bowel bleeding. *Gastrointest Endosc* 2017;85(1):22–31.

ASGE Technology Committee, Parsi MA, Schulman AR, et al. Devices for endoscopic hemostasis of nonvariceal GI bleeding (with videos). *Gastrointest Endosc* 2019;4(7):285–99.

Garcia-Tsao G, Abraldes JG, Berzigotti A, et al. Portal hypertensive bleeding in cirrhosis: Risk stratification, diagnosis, and management: 2016 practice guidance by the American Association for the Study of Liver Diseases. *Hepatology* 2017;65(1):310–335.

Gralnek IM, Stanley AJ, Morris AJ, et al. Endoscopic diagnosis and management of nonvariceal upper gastrointestinal hemorrhage (NVUGIH): European Society of Gastrointestinal Endoscopy (ESGE) Guideline—Update 2021. *Endoscopy* 2021;53(3):300–32.

Henry Z, Patel K, Patton H, et al. AGA clinical practice update on management of bleeding gastric varices: Expert review. *Clin Gastroenterol Hepatol* 2021;19(6):1098–1107.

Karstensen JG, Ebigbo A, Bhat P, et al. Endoscopic treatment of variceal upper gastrointestinal bleeding: European Society of Gastrointestinal Endoscopy (ESGE) Cascade Guideline. *Endosc Int Open* 2020;8(7):E990–E997.

Laine L, Barkun AN, Saltzman JR, et al. ACG Clinical Guideline: Upper gastrointestinal and ulcer bleeding. *Am J Gastroenterol* 2021;116(5):899–917.

Mullady DK, Wang AY, Waschke KA. AGA clinical practice update on endoscopic therapies for non-variceal upper gastrointestinal bleeding: Expert review. *Gastroenterology* 2020;159(3):1120–8.

Esophageal

Adler DG, Siddiqui AA. Endoscopic management of esophageal strictures. *Gastrointest Endosc* 2017;86(1):35–43.

ASGE Standards of Practice Committee, Qumseya B, Sultan S, et al. ASGE guideline on screening and surveillance of Barrett's esophagus. *Gastrointest Endosc* 2019;90(3):335–59.

Brindise E, Khashab MA, El Abiad R. Insights into the endoscopic management of esophageal achalasia. *Ther Adv Gastrointest Endosc* 2021;14:26317745211014706.

Spaander MCW, van der Bogt RD, Baron TH, et al. Esophageal stenting for benign and malignant disease: European Society of Gastrointestinal Endoscopy (ESGE) Guideline—Update 2021. *Endoscopy* 2021;53(7):751–62.

General

ASGE Technology Committee, Diehl DL, Adler DG, et al. Endoscopic retrieval devices. *Gastrointest Endosc* 2009;69(6):997–1003.

ASGE Technology Committee, Hwang JH, Konda V, et al. Endoscopic mucosal resection. *Gastrointest Endosc* 2015;82(2):215–26.

ASGE Technology Committee, Tokar JL, Barth JL, et al. Electrosurgical generators. *Gastrointest Endosc* 2015;78(2):197–208.

ASGE Training Committee, Aihara H, Kushnir V, et al. Core curriculum for endoscopic mucosal resection. *Gastrointest Endosc* 2021;93(2):293–6.

Bai Y, Yang F, Liu C. Expert consensus on the clinical application of high-frequency electrosurgery in digestive endoscopy (2020, Shanghai). *J Dig Dis* 2022;23(1):2–12.

Bounds BC. Endoscopic retrieval devices. *Tech Gastrointest Endosc* 2006;8(1):16–21.

Farin G, Grund KE. Principles of electrosurgery, laser, and argon plasma coagulation with particular regard to endoscopy. In: Cotton, PB, eds. *Advanced Digestive Endoscopy: Practice and Safety*. Malden, MA: Blackwell Publishing, 2008:101–29.

Lee JH, Kedia P, Stavropoulos SN, et al. AGA clinical practice update on endoscopic management of perforations in gastrointestinal tract: Expert review. *Clin Gastroenterol Hepatol* 2021;19(11):2252–61.

Morris ML, Tucker RD, Baron TH, et al. Electrosurgery in gastrointestinal endoscopy: Principles to practice. *Am J Gastroenterol* 2009;104(6):1563–74.

Vitale DS, Wang K, Jamil LH, et al. Endoscopic mucosal resection in children. *J Pediatr Gastroenterol Nutr* 2022;74(1):20–4.

CHAPTER 7

Colonoscopy and Flexible Sigmoidoscopy

History

The history of colonoscopy started in 1958 in Japan with Matsunaga's intracolonic use of the gastrocamera and then Niwa's development of the "sigmocamera" (Video 7.1). Following Hirschowitz's development of the fiberoptic bundle in 1957–1960 for use in side-viewing gastroscopes, Overholt in the United States performed the first fiberoptic flexible sigmoidoscopy in 1963 and introduced a commercial forward-viewing short "fiberoptic coloscope" in 1966 (American Cystoscope Manufacturers Inc.). Others used passive fiberoptic viewing bundles or side-viewing gastroscopes guided up the colon radiologically or pulled up by a swallowed transintestinal "guide string and pulley" system. By 1969 Japanese firms (Olympus Optical and Machida) offered remarkably effective colonoscopes, with precise two-way angulation and a torque-stable shaft, though fragility of Japanese glass fibers restricted angulation to around 90° and the angle of view was limited to 70°.

Gastric snare polypectomy was first described by Niwa in Japan in 1968–9 and snaring of colon polyps was pioneered in 1971 by Deyhle in Europe and Shinya in the United States. In the mid-1970s four-way acutely angulating instruments were introduced, and in 1983 the video endoscope arrived (Welch-Allyn). Although colonoscope production has continued in the United States, Germany, and China, major Japanese camera manufacturers continue to dominate the market. Other innovative video-colonoscopes are also emerging.

Indications and limitations, and alternatives

The place of colonoscopy in clinical practice depends on local circumstances and available endoscopic expertise. Although colonoscopy has been considered the gold standard exam, its expense, technical demands, and occasional adverse events can make alternative technologies attractive for whole-colon examination of

Cotton and Williams' Practical Gastrointestinal Endoscopy: The Fundamentals, Eighth Edition.
Catharine M. Walsh, Ahmir Ahmad, Brian P. Saunders, Jonathan Cohen, Peter B. Cotton, and Christopher B. Williams.
© 2024 John Wiley & Sons Ltd. Published 2024 by John Wiley & Sons Ltd.
Companion website: www.wiley.com/go/cottonwilliams8e

Table 7.1 Colonoscopy: indications and yield

High-yield indications	Low-yield indications
Anemia/bleeding/occult blood loss	Constipation, acute or chronic
Persistent diarrhea	Abdominal distension or flatulence
Inflammatory disease assessment	Abdominal pain alone
Genetic cancer risk	
Abnormality on imaging	
Therapy	

some "low-yield" or high-risk patients. Similarly, on the grounds of logistics, safety, and patient acceptability, flexible sigmoidoscopy is validated for population screening as well as its diagnostic role in clinically selected patients with anorectal symptoms.

Colonoscopy and flexible sigmoidoscopy achieve more than radiological imaging techniques do because of their greater accuracy and histologic and therapeutic capabilities. Color view and biopsy makes total colonoscopy particularly relevant to patients with bleeding, anemia, bowel frequency, or diarrhea. Flexible sigmoidoscopy alone may be sufficient for some patients, such as those with left iliac fossa pain or bright red per-rectal bleeding. Because of enhanced accuracy and therapy, colonoscopy is preferred for any patient at increased risk of cancer—in whom detection and removal of all adenomas is important to prevent cancer and as a predictor of long-term cancer risk. Colonoscopy is thus the method of choice for many clinical indications and for cancer surveillance examinations and follow-up (Table 7.1). Endoscopy is also particularly useful in the postoperative patient, either to inspect in close-up (and biopsy if necessary) any deformity at the anastomosis or to avoid difficulties for the radiologist of achieving adequate distension in patients with a stoma.

Scanning techniques

Computerized tomography (CT) colonography has replaced double-contrast barium enema (DCBE) as the radiological investigation of choice for the colon, with the advantages of being quicker and more available than the magnetic resonance (MR) alternative. Scanning requires technical expertise from the radiographer performing it and obsessional care by the radiologist interpreting the results. A few patients who are very difficult to colonoscope for reasons of anatomy or postoperative adhesions may be best examined by combining limited left-sided colonoscopy with CT colonography to demonstrate the proximal colon. CT colonography has the advantage that it can be performed before or after colonoscopy and with the same bowel preparation, although the majority of scanning procedures are now best performed with "fecal tagging" using water-soluble contrast agents. MR colonography is rarely used apart from in younger patients or those concerned about radiation exposure.

Combined procedures

The combination of two diagnostic procedures (colonoscopy and virtual colonography) is rarely necessary unless the colonoscopy is incomplete or when assessing an area of bowel wall thickening. Standard-sized pinch biopsies at colonoscopy do not preclude immediate CT colonography but caution is required if a larger polyp resection with electrosurgery (diathermy) has taken place due to a possible increased risk of perforation from subsequent gas distension and a weakened bowel wall.

Limitations of colonoscopy

• *Incomplete examination* can be due to inadequate bowel preparation, uncontrollable looping, severe bowel fixation and angulation due to diverticulosis or pelvic adhesions, an obstructing lesion, or inadequate operator skills. Unless the ileo-cecal valve is reached and photodocumented with clear views of the cecal pole, completion has not been proved.

• *Gross errors in colonoscopic localization and "blind spots" are possible* even for expert endoscopists. Blind areas, with the possibility of missing even large lesions, occur especially in the cecum (particularly behind the ileo-cecal valve), recto-sigmoid junction, around any acute bends such as at the flexures, and also in the rectal ampulla. The latest high-definition, high-resolution video endoscopic systems and monitors *and tip-mounted accessories such as cuffs and caps can improve the view* but colonoscopic examination, even rigorously performed, probably only achieves 90% accuracy for detection of small lesions. This recognized "miss rate" should always be explained as part of the patient consent process. Artificial intelligence systems can also help in polyp detection but are only effective when the mucosal surface is revealed to the endoscope camera.

Hazards and adverse events

Colonoscopy, despite its virtues, is more hazardous than diagnostic alternatives (currently around one perforation per 2,000 colonoscopic examinations, compared with perforations in 1:25,000 CT colonography exams). Unskilled endoscopists needing to use heavy sedation or general anesthesia to cover up ineptitude are likely to run greater risks. It should, therefore, not be regarded as failure to abandon a tough colonoscopy in favor of immediate CT colonography, as "pressing on regardless" could result in an avoidable perforation and subsequent sequelae.

Instrument shaft or tip perforations

Colonoscopy perforations are usually caused by inexperienced users and the use of excessive force when pushing in or pulling out. In a pathologically fixed, severely ulcerated, or necrotic colon, however, forces that would be safe in a normal colon may be hazardous. Either the tip of the instrument or a loop formed by its shaft can perforate. Shaft loop perforations are characteristically larger than expected, so, if in doubt, surgery should be advised. On the other hand, post-procedure peritoneal symptoms can sometimes be managed conservatively (see "Management following adverse events" below). Surgery performed soon after apparently uneventful colonoscopy can show small tears in the ante-mesenteric serosal aspect of the colon and hematomas in the mesentery. In rare cases the spleen has been avulsed during straightening maneuvers when the tip is hooked around the splenic flexure.

Air pressure perforations

These include "blow-outs" of diverticula and ileo-cecal perforation following colonoscopy limited to the sigmoid colon due to displaced gas and barotrauma. Surprisingly high gas pressures result if the scope tip is impacted in a diverticulum or if insufflation is excessive, for instance when trying to distend and pass a stricture or segment of severe diverticular disease. Use of water-assisted insertion and CO_2 insufflation minimizes these serious risks. CO_2 is rapidly reabsorbed post-procedure with significantly less patient discomfort and has now almost completely replaced the use of room air for gas distension during colonoscopy. Diverticula are thin-walled and have also been perforated with biopsy forceps or by the instrument tip. It is surprisingly easy to confuse a large diverticular orifice with the bowel lumen or to mistakenly identify an inverted diverticulum, usually in the proximal colon, as a small sessile polyp.

Hypotensive episodes

Hypotensive episodes, even cardiac or respiratory arrest, can be provoked by the combination of oversedation with the intense vagal stimulus of forceful or prolonged colonoscopy.

Hypoxia

Hypoxia is more likely in elderly patients sensitive to intravenous sedation but should be a thing of the past if pulse oximetry (or CO_2 capnography) is routinely used and nasal oxygen given prophylactically to all sedated patients.

Infection

As mentioned elsewhere, prophylactic antibiotics are rarely indicated before colonoscopy, then only for well-defined groups such as severely immunocompromised patients and possibly those with ascites or on peritoneal dialysis. However, Gram-negative septicemia can result from instrumentation (especially in neonates or the elderly) and unexplained post-procedure pyrexia or collapse should be investigated with blood cultures and managed appropriately.

Management following adverse events

Therapeutic procedures inevitably increase the risk of adverse events, including dilatations, electrocoagulation of bleeding points, or sessile polypectomies. However, the hazards are remarkably infrequent compared with the morbidity and mortality considered acceptable for surgery. To generalize (and perhaps exaggerate), endoscopic misadventure risks surgery; surgical misadventure risks death. The endoscopist should therefore be on guard for problems that can occur and should only undertake therapeutic procedures with the knowledge of a back-up surgical team.

It is worth remembering that fatalities have also been reported after colonoscopic perforation followed by unnecessary surgery (rather than relying on endoscopic management or conservative management with antibiotic cover). The decision whether or not to operate after an adverse event can be a subtle one, but the maxim should be "if in doubt, operate"—although the surgeon consulted needs to be aware of the particular endoscopic circumstances. Most therapeutic perforations will be small and occur in a well-prepared colon; therefore, early recognition and endoscopic repair are often possible with through-the-scope or over-the-scope clips. Delayed intraperitoneal perforations, once peritonitis is established, will usually require surgery. Close clinical review in combination with appropriate timing of CT scanning are the key to successful management of colonoscopic perforations.

Safety

Safety during colonoscopy comes from gentle technique. Before starting a colonoscopy, it is impossible to know if there are adhesions, whether the bowel is easily distensible, and whether its mesenteries are free-floating or fixed; pain or increased resistance from the scope tip are the warning signs that the bowel or its attachments are being unreasonably strained. The endoscopist should respect any protest from the patient; a mild groan in a sedated patient may be equivalent to a scream of pain without sedation. If propofol or deep sedation is used, the endoscopist must be even more cautious when resistance on the scope shaft or tip is encountered, as the early warning of impending bowel injury from patient discomfort is eliminated. If there is concern, the endoscopist should be prepared to change approach and use a smaller-diameter scope, a balloon endoscope system, or revert to a CT colonography. *Total colonoscopy is not always technically possible, even for experts.*

Despite its potential hazards, skilled colonoscopy is amazingly safe; it is certainly justified by its clinical yield and the high morbidity of colonic surgery (which would often be the therapeutic alternative). For the less skilled endoscopist, partnership with CT colonography in "difficult" cases should reduce the risks—with re-referral to an expert endoscopist if pathology is found.

Informed consent

Obtaining full informed patient consent is essential before an invasive procedure such as colonoscopy, with its potential for adverse events. The patient should understand the rationale for undergoing the procedure, its benefits, risks, limitations, and alternatives, and be given written information to digest in advance as well as have an opportunity to ask any questions—ideally a pre-procedure meeting. Chapter 4 is relevant and has a sample colonoscopy information leaflet (Fig 4.2).

If a child is unable to provide informed consent themselves (e.g. they are too young), they should still be provided basic information about the procedure and asked to assent to the procedure (i.e. express their agreement), and informed consent should be obtained from a designated parent or guardian, consistent with local law.

Precise approaches to the explanation of risks vary from country to country and should be tailored to some extent to the perceived insights and anxieties of the individual patient. Some patients wish to know everything, whereas some would be distressed to have scary and unlikely minutiae (such as "the unlikely possibility of death") spelled out to them. Any possible adverse event with an incidence greater than 1:100 or with potentially serious consequences such as perforation should be explained. A frank discussion of the "pluses and minuses" of anticipated therapeutic procedures, such as removal of large sessile polyps or dilation of strictures, should be mandatory. Ideally, the endoscopist should quote personal figures and experience.

It is logical and our routine practice to mention to all adult patients the possibility of post-polypectomy delayed bleeding occurring for up to 14 days post-procedure, in case a polyp is found incidentally during colonoscopy and is judged to require removal (even though the procedure is scheduled as "diagnostic"). Most patients will acquiesce immediately, but a commonsense discussion of practicalities is relevant. A patient about to have a holiday in remote parts or organizing a family wedding or other major event may be disinclined to take any risk whatsoever—and would justifiably be aggrieved should an adverse event occur. A final important part to the consent process is to explain that it is possible to miss polyps or, rarely, even early cancers during the examination and also that if new or unusual symptoms develop after an apparently normal colonoscopy the patient should still seek medical advice.

Contraindications and infective hazards

There are few patients in whom colonoscopy is contraindicated. Any patient who might otherwise be considered for diagnostic laparotomy because of colonic disease is fit for colonoscopy, and colonoscopy is often undertaken in very high-risk cases in the hope of avoiding surgery.

• *There is no absolute contraindication to colonoscopy during pregnancy*, although it might be best avoided in those with a history of miscarriage.

• *There is no contraindication to the examination of infected patients* (e.g. patients with infectious diarrhea or hepatitis) because all normal organisms and viruses should be inactivated by routine cleaning and disinfection procedures (see Chapter 3).

• *Antibiotic prophylaxis is unnecessary*, according to current United Kingdom and United States guidelines, even after heart valve replacement or previous bacterial endocarditis. It may be indicated in severely immunocompromised patients (see Chapter 4).

BUT

• *Colonoscopy is absolutely contraindicated* during, and for 2–3 weeks after, *acute diverticulitis*, due to the risk of perforation from a localized abscess or cavity. It should not be performed, or only with the greatest care and minimal insufflation, in any patient with marked *abdominal tenderness, peritonism, or peritonitis*.

• *Colonoscopy should only be undertaken with good reason and extreme care when there is severe inflammation* (ulcerative, Crohn's, or ischemic colitis), especially if abdominal tenderness suggests an increased risk of perforation. If large and deep ulcers are seen it may be wise to limit or abandon the examination. After irradiation, especially a year or more after exposure, narrowed or obstructed bowel can be perforated without using excessive force. If insertion proves difficult it may be best to withdraw or to change to a smaller instrument.

• *Colonoscopy is relatively contraindicated* for 3 months after *myocardial infarction*, when it is unwise owing to the risk of dysrhythmias.

• *Colonoscopy is relatively contraindicated in patients with known ascites or on peritoneal dialysis* because of the probability of scope pressure causing transient release of bowel organisms into the bloodstream and peritoneal cavity.

• *Other factors can be relevant* and should be considered during the process of obtaining information and consent, including previous medical history and current medications. For obvious reasons, medications such as anticoagulants or insulin may affect management. A cardiac pacemaker theoretically contraindicates use of magnetic endoscope imaging or argon plasma coagulation (APC), but these should not affect modern insulated pacemakers. Patients with implantable defibrillators, however, are at risk from inappropriate firing of their devices during standard electrosurgery. These patients require full cardiac monitoring during electrosurgery, with a technician available to switch off the device before and turn it on after the procedure.

Patient preparation

Most patients can manage bowel preparation at home, arrive for colonoscopy, and walk out shortly afterwards. Management routines depend on national, organizational, and individual factors. Overall management is influenced, among other things, by:

• cost
• facilities available
• type of bowel preparation and sedation used
• age and co-morbidity of the individual patient
• potential for major therapeutic procedures
• availability of adequate facilities and nursing staff for day-care and recovery.

Experienced colonoscopists in private practice or large units are motivated to organize streamlined day-case routines, even for patients with large polyps. Sedation practices for colonoscopy vary widely throughout the world and ideally the sedation needs of a patient are ascertained in advance of the scheduled procedure. For routine procedures many adult patients choose no sedation, given the advantage of rapid recovery afterwards and the ability to drive and go back to work the same day. Others will prefer deeper sedation and, increasingly, small doses of titrated propofol are used to augment short-acting opioid analgesia. Propofol has a very short half-life (1–2 minutes), which means that once it is stopped patients recover very quickly; this helps maintain rapid turnaround within busy endoscopy units. However, deeper sedation (with propofol or higher doses of midazolam) does risk respiratory compromise and necessitates the presence of an anesthetist or specialist anesthetic-trained practitioner. A deeply sedated patient during colonoscopy is more difficult to reposition and pain feedback is diminished, so extreme care is required when some degree of force is required during insertion. However, a more comfortable procedure can be assured, particularly for children, those with difficult anatomy, and for longer therapeutic procedures where the endoscopist can focus entirely without being distracted by the sedation needs of a restless patient.

Colonoscopy can be made quick and easy for the majority of patients. This requires both a properly planned day-care facility and an endoscopist with the confidence and skill to work gently and reasonably fast. Some flexibility of approach is wise. Very few patients are better admitted before or after the procedure. The very young or old, sick, or very constipated may need professional supervision during bowel preparation. Frail patients may merit overnight observation afterwards if their domestic circumstances are not supportive or they live far away. We do rarely admit a few patients for polypectomy, especially if the lesion is very large and sessile and the patient has a bleeding diathesis or is unavoidably on anticoagulants or antiplatelet medications (clopidogrel, etc.). Even such patients, however, providing they live near good medical support services and have been fully informed about what to do in a crisis, can often be justifiably managed on an outpatient basis, as adverse events are rare and can in any case be "delayed" several days post-procedure. We always provide the patient with a copy of their report when they leave the endoscopy unit, and this contains information on symptoms to look out for that might herald an adverse event and emergency contact numbers should they have any problems. Patients are clearly informed that there is a risk of delayed bleeding, particularly after polypectomy involving electro-surgery, and also, that they should not undergo long-haul flights in the 14 days post-procedure in case a delayed bleed occurred while they were airborne.

Bowel preparation

An informed team member should be available to talk to the patient at the time of booking to explain the procedure, including the importance of successful bowel preparation—although printed instructions and explanations will be sufficient for most patients. The majority of patients find that the worst part of colonoscopy is the bowel preparation and that the anticipation of the procedure (including fear of indignity, a painful experience, and/or the possible findings) is much worse than the reality of the colonoscopy itself. Minutes spent in explanation and motivation may prevent a prolonged, unpleasant, and inaccurate examination due to bad preparation. The patient needs to know that a properly prepared colon is the single most important factor for a successful colonoscopy.

Written dietary instructions are well worthwhile, as many patients, anxious to get a good result, find it easier to follow specific instructions "to the letter." Clear instructions avoid unnecessary anxieties and many telephone calls. Bowel preparation apps, text reminders, and online instructions and videos can also be a useful addition.

Limited preparation

Enemas alone are usually effective for limited colonoscopy or flexible sigmoidoscopy in the "normal" colon. The patient need not diet and typically has one or two disposable phosphate enemas (e.g. Fleet Phospho-soda®, Micralax®), self-administered or given by nursing staff. Examination can be performed shortly after evacuation occurs—usually within 10–15 minutes—so that there is no time for more proximal bowel contents to descend. The colon can often be perfectly prepared to the transverse colon in younger subjects. Phosphate enemas, however, should not be used in babies as they are contraindicated due to the risk of hyperphosphatemia. Note that patients with any tendency to faint or with functional bowel symptoms (pain, flatulence, etc.) are more likely to have vasovagal problems after stimulant enemas; make sure they are supervised or have a call button. Lavatory doors should be able to be opened from and toward the outside in case the patient should faint against the door.

Diverticular disease or stricturing requires full bowel preparation even for a limited examination, because bowel preparation will be less effective and enemas less likely to work.

If obstruction is a possibility, per-oral preparation is dangerous, even potentially fatal. In ileus or "pseudo-obstruction" normal preparation simply does not work. One or more large-volume enemas are administered in such circumstances (up to 1 L or more can be held by most colons). A dose of bisacodyl can be added to the enema to improve evacuation (see "Magnesium salts" below).

Full preparation

The object of full preparation is to cleanse the whole colon, especially the proximal parts, which are characteristically coated with surface residue after limited regimens. However, patients and colons vary. No single preparation regime predictably suits every patient, and it is often necessary to be prepared to adapt to individual needs. Constipated patients need extra preparation; those with severe colitis may be unfit to have anything other than a warm saline or tap water enema. A preparation that has previously proved unpalatable, made the patient vomit, or that failed is unlikely to be a success on another occasion—a different one should be substituted. Current data support "split-dose" administration (see "Routine for taking oral preparation" below) to increase acceptability and resultant success of preparation.

Dietary restriction is a crucial part of preparation. The patient should have no indigestible or high-residue food for 72 hours before colonoscopy (avoiding muesli, fibrous vegetables, seeds, mushrooms, fruit, nuts, raisins, etc.). Staying on clear fluids for 24 hours is even better if the patient is compliant but is not really necessary and may affect compliance. Soft foods that are easily digested (soups, omelets, potato without the skin, cheese, and ice cream) can be eaten up to (and including) lunch on the day preceding colonoscopy. Only supper and breakfast before colonoscopy need to be replaced with fluids. For most nonsedated or lightly sedated procedures, fluids, including plain tea or coffee can be drunk up to the last minute, since minor fluid residues present no problem to the endoscopist. However, if the procedure is planned with deep sedation, then the patient should be nil by mouth for at least 2 hours prior to the procedure to reduce any risk of aspiration.

Drink extra clear fluids—the more the better! Fruit-flavored or isotonic drinks are found by many to be easier to drink in large quantities than water. Any other clear drink, water ices or sorbets (not black currant), consommé (hot or cold), boiled sweets, or peppermints can all help to vary the preparation regimen and improve compliance. There is no reason why anyone should feel ravenous or unduly deprived of calories by the time of colonoscopy.

Medications or supplements containing iron should be stopped at least 7 days before colonoscopy, as organic iron tannates produce an inky black and viscous stool, which interferes with inspection and is difficult to clear. *Constipating agents* should also be stopped 5 days before.

Most medications can be continued as usual, except for modification of anticoagulant regimens and withdrawal of clopidogrel and similar platelet-inhibiting agents for 1 week before planned polypectomy. Aspirin in low dose is usually continued as there is no increased risk of post-polypectomy bleeding.

PEG–electrolyte preparation

Balanced electrolyte solution with polyethylene glycol solution (PEG) is very widely used. This is primarily because it has formal approval from the US Food and Drug Administration (FDA) (e.g. GoLYTELY®, NuLYTELY®, CoLyte®, KleenPrep®, Plenvu®, etc.) and comes with suitable flavorings, convenient packaging, and is easily prescribed, but it is surprisingly expensive. Although the PEG component of a PEG-electrolyte mixture contributes to the majority of the packaged weight, volume, and expense, it results in only a minority of the osmolality (sodium salts being, of physiological necessity, the important component). Even chilled, its taste is mildly unpleasant due to the Na_2SO_4, bicarbonate, and KCl included to minimize body fluxes. Modification of the original formula by omitting Na_2SO_4 and reducing KCl only slightly improves the taste. Many patients find the 4 liter volume of traditional PEG-electrolyte solutions difficult to tolerate and ingest and this has led to further modifications to reduce the overall volume required for adequate cleansing. MoviPrep®, which combines PEG-electrolyte with ascorbic acid (aspartame, the sweetening agent used in it, can be nauseating to some patients) is made up to 2 liters and Plenvu® increases the dose of ascorbic acid to create a 1 liter preparation. However, to avoid dehydration it is recommended that at least 1 liter of additional fluid is taken with both MoviPrep® and Plenvu®. A low-volume preparation raises the possibility of taking it all in the morning for afternoon or evening colonoscopy appointments, with significant time savings for the patient and less time off work.

Patient acceptance of all PEG-electrolyte-based oral preparations can be enhanced by chilling the solutions or drinking them via a straw, which dulls the salty/sweet aftertaste. There are conflicting reports about whether the addition of prokinetic agents or laxatives improves results; the consensus is that it does not.

Magnesium salts

Magnesium citrate and other magnesium salts are very poorly absorbed, acting as an "osmotic purge." The gently cathartic properties of "spa" waters rich in magnesium salts, such as Vichy water, have been known since Roman times. Picolax® or Pico-Salax®, a proprietary combination, produces both magnesium citrate (from magnesium oxide and citric acid) and bisacodyl (from bacterial action on sodium picosulfate). It tastes acceptable and works well in most patients. Taking two to three bisacodyl tablets in addition improves results but can cause cramping.

Routine for taking oral preparation

Low-residue diet instructions should have been followed, ideally for several days in the case of those with known constipation or slow transit. The patient should apply a barrier cream to avoid perianal soreness (colorless to avoid endoscope lens contamination as the scope is inserted through the anus). The evening before colonoscopy will be fluid-dominated—input and output—so social events should not be scheduled but there will be plenty of time for watching television or reading between "calls."

As mentioned previously, large-volume solutions are ideally split-administered in two doses, starting on the afternoon or evening before, but *it is essential that some oral preparation is taken on the morning of the examination* so that cecal contents remain fluid and easily aspirated.

The patient should be encouraged to carry on with normal activities, rather than sitting still during the drinking period; exercise stimulates transit and evacuation. Bowel actions should start within 1–3 hours but can be much delayed in constipated patients or those who prove to have a long colon.

Bowel preparation in special circumstances
Children

Bowel preparation can pose a challenge in the pediatric population. An ideal preparation is one that is low volume, palatable, inexpensive, and effective without adverse events. Children under 2 years of age may be almost completely prepared with clear liquids for 24 hours plus a normal saline enema (5 mL/kg). For children over 2 years of age, bowel preparation can be accomplished with intestinal lavage using osmotic agents, such as PEG with and without electrolytes, stimulant laxatives, such as senna and bisacodyl, and/or enemas. Of note, phosphate enemas are recognized to cause potentially fatal adverse events including electrolyte shifts and hyperphosphatemia so are contraindicated in young children and generally not recommended in anyone under 18 years of age.

PEG-3350 preparations without electrolytes (e.g. Miralax®, RestoraLAX®) that are mixed with commercially available sports drinks are increasingly used for bowel preparation in children, at doses as much as 10 times higher than those recommended for the standard treatment of constipation. Sodium picosulfate with magnesium citrate (Pico-Salax®) mixed with a small volume of fluid is also commonly used, where available, in split doses 8–12 hours apart (0.25, 0.5, and 1 sachet/dose for children <6, 6–12, and >12 years old). Additional fluid is required for the preparation to work effectively and prevent dehydration. PEG-electrolyte solutions can also be used at a dose of 20–40 mL/kg/hour (maximum 1 L/hour) over 4 hours; however, these are often not well tolerated, and most children require admission for nasogastric tube administration.

Colitis patients

Patients with colitis require special care, during and after preparation. The principal indication for colonoscopy in adult patients with inflammatory bowel disease is cancer surveillance, particularly for those with longstanding extensive disease. These patients may be more difficult to prepare for colonoscopy and extended bowel preparation should be considered (see "Constipated patients" below). Patients attending for surveillance colonoscopy should be in remission as active inflammation causes the mucosal lining to be sticky and difficult to prepare adequately for detailed mucosal visualization.

Relapses of inflammatory bowel disease occasionally occur after overvigorous bowel preparation, but balanced PEG-electrolyte solutions are well tolerated. A simple tap water or saline enema will clear the distal colon sufficiently for limited colonoscopy. Patients with severe colitis are unlikely to need colonoscopy at all, as plain abdominal X-ray, ultrasonography, or scanning will usually give enough information.

For severely ill patients, any distension is risky and colonoscopy is positively contraindicated due to the potential for perforation. When the indication for colonoscopy in a colitis patient is to exclude cancer or to reach the terminal ileum to help in differential diagnosis, full and vigorous preparation is necessary.

Constipated patients

Patients with constipation typically need extended bowel preparation with additional bowel preparation given over a longer time period, as transit is often delayed. A standard extra prep regimen would involve two doses of MoviPrep® early afternoon and evening the day before and an additional dose on the morning of the procedure. Full bowel evacuation is very difficult to achieve in patients with true megacolon or Hirschsprung's disease, in whom colonoscopy should be avoided if at all possible. Constipated patients should have at least 48 hours on a low-residue diet, as they normally take a high-fiber regime but have slow transit. They should continue any habitually taken purgatives in addition to the regime for colonoscopy preparation.

Colostomy patients

Colostomy patients are as difficult to prepare as normal subjects. Oral preparation is well tolerated, whereas enemas/colostomy washouts are tedious and difficult for nursing staff to perform satisfactorily, unless the patient is accustomed to this and can do it for themselves.

Stomas, pouches, and ileo-rectal anastomoses present few problems. Ileostomies are self-emptying and normally need no preparation other than perhaps a few hours of fasting and clear fluid intake. Ileo-anal pelvic pouches can be managed either by saline or phosphate enema or by reduced volume of oral lavage. After ileo-rectal anastomosis, the small intestine can adapt and enlarge to an amazing degree within some months of surgery, so that if the object of the examination is to examine the small intestine, full oral preparation should be given. For a limited look, any conventional enema is usually enough (NB stimulant enemas sometimes cause a vasovagal response).

Defunctioned bowel, for instance the distal loop of a "double-barreled" colostomy, always contains a considerable amount of viscid mucus and inspissated cell debris, which will block the colonoscope. Conventional tap water or saline rectal enemas or tube lavage through the colostomy are needed to clear a defunctioned bowel. Hypertonic (phosphate) or stimulant enemas will be less effective.

Colonic bleeding

Active colonic bleeding helps preparation, as blood is a good purgative. Some patients requiring emergency colonoscopy may need no specific preparation at all, providing that examination is started during the phase of active bright red bleeding. Position change during insertion of the instrument will shift the blood and create an air interface through which the instrument can be passed. Changing to the right lateral position clears the proximal sigmoid and descending colon, which is otherwise a blood-filled sump.

For hemodynamically unstable or shocked patients, CT angiography is the quickest and least invasive means of localizing the site of blood loss. If positive, the lesion should be treated with interventional radiology (IR) or endoscopically. If treatment fails, an alternative endoscopic treatment modality or surgery may be required. If IR is successful, an inpatient lower GI endoscopic procedure should be organized. Where the CT angiogram is negative, a colonoscopy with bowel preparation should be organized for the next available list.

Actively bleeding patients requiring preparation for more accurate total colonoscopy can be managed by nasogastric tube lavage, which allows examination within an hour or two and ensures that blood is washed out distal to the bleeding point, rather than carried proximally with enemas. Blood can be refluxed to the terminal ileum from a left colon source, which makes localization difficult unless it is being constantly washed downward by a per-oral high-volume preparation. Massively bleeding patients can be examined per-operatively with on-table colon lavage combining a cecostomy tube with a large-bore rectal suction tube (and bucket), but more often should be managed angiographically with no preparation at all.

Medication

Attitudes toward medication differ greatly from country to country. We favor adapting to the individual patient.

Sedation and analgesia

All aspects of the procedure, including the medication options, should be explained when the colonoscopy booking is arranged. The patient should receive preliminary verbal and written explanation about bowel preparation and what to expect of the procedure (whether from a doctor or nurse). At this point some patients may judge that they want full medication, others that they will hope to work normally or to drive afterwards. On arrival for colonoscopy, a few minutes of further explanation will reassure and calm most patients and allow the endoscopist to judge whether the particular individual is likely to require sedation and, if so, how much. Most people tolerate some discomfort without resentment if they understand the reason for it. Few people expect to be semi-anesthetized for a visit to the dentist, but on the other hand they understandably expect the intensity and duration of any discomfort to be within "acceptable limits." Pain thresholds and individual attitudes to pain are not always easy to predict before colonoscopy, because tolerance of the (peculiarly unpleasant) quality of visceral pain varies so much. It is sensible to warn the patient that there will be a few seconds of "wind" or a transient sensation of "urgency."

During a typical and correctly performed colonoscopy, minor discomfort may be experienced by the patient (after prior warning) only briefly for one or two occasions during the procedure. Using moderate or no sedation, and employing the skills, changes of position, water infusion, and other "tricks of the trade" described in this chapter, pain only occurs during looping in the sigmoid colon and while passing the sigmoid-descending colon junction. During the rest of an uncomplicated procedure a patient with an average pain threshold should experience little more than mild distension or the urge to pass flatus. It is worth pointing out to the patient that pain is useful to the endoscopist because it shows that a loop is forming, but is not dangerous and can usually be stopped in a few seconds (by straightening out the loop that is causing it).

The use of sedation has advantages and disadvantages. The unsedated or very lightly sedated patient can cooperate by changing position, needs no recovery period, and can travel home unaided immediately. The colonoscopist is also encouraged to develop dexterous and gentle insertion technique. On the other hand, some patients are very anxious and have low pain thresholds, leading to an unpleasant or failed procedure. If light "conscious sedation" is used (typically equivalent in effect to two to three glasses of wine or beer), the patient is likely to find the examination tolerable or to have amnesia for it. The endoscopist is helped to be thorough by the knowledge that the patient is comfortable, and is also more likely to achieve total colonoscopy in a shorter time. Using heavy sedation, endoscopists can get away with ham-handed and forcibly looping technique—a bad investment in the long term, less likely to achieve complete examinations, more likely to result in adverse events, and more expensive in instrument repair bills.

It is often said that it is dangerous to sedate because the safety factor of pain is removed. This is not strictly true, providing that the endoscopist's threshold of awareness lowers as the patient's pain threshold is raised—taking restlessness or changes of facial expression as a warning that tissues and attachments are being overstretched.

Most endoscopists who perform procedures in adults use a balanced approach to sedation that will be affected by many factors, including personal experience and the individual patient's attitude. A relaxed patient with a short colon having a limited examination rarely needs sedation, but an anxious patient with a tortuous colon, severe diverticular disease, or a bad previous experience may need deep sedation and benefit from water infusion technique. Patients with irritable bowel syndrome or pain as presenting features are likely to be hypersensitive to stretch and will similarly benefit from opiates or deep sedation with propofol and water infusion. Currently, most pediatric endoscopic procedures involve anesthesiologist-directed sedation.

Nitrous oxide inhalation

Nitrous oxide/oxygen (e.g. Entonox®) inhalation can be a useful alternative to intravenous sedation/analgesia, is short acting, and permits the patient to drive 30 minutes after the procedure. Contraindications include any situation where inhaled gas might collect within an enclosed body cavity such as those with known large bullae from emphysema, small bowel obstruction, middle ear surgery, and/or prior retinal surgery involving the creation of an intraocular gas bubble as well as those at risk of pneumothorax. The 50:50 nitrous oxide/oxygen mixture is self-administered by the patient, inhaled from a small cylinder fitted with a demand valve. Breathing the gas through a small single-use mouthpiece (Fig 7.1) avoids the difficulties that can be experienced in getting a good fit with a face mask and mitigates the phobia that some patients experience with masks.

The patient is shown how to inhale, then "pre-breathes" for a minute or two as the endoscopist prepares to start the procedure,

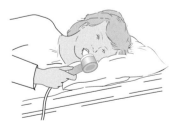

Fig 7.1 Nitrous oxide/oxygen mixture is breathed through a mouthpiece.

with the intention of achieving gas saturation of the body fatty tissues. Thereafter it takes only 20–30 seconds of gas breathing, when required, to obtain a "high" that makes short-lived pain more tolerable. Nitrous oxide/oxygen inhalation should prove useful for some flexible sigmoidoscopies and, when used alone, can be sufficient for motivated patients having total colonoscopy by a skilled endoscopist. Scared patients, prolonged or difficult examinations, and examinations by inexpert endoscopists require conventional sedation.

Moderate sedation

The ideal moderate sedation for colonoscopy would last only 5–10 minutes, with a strong analgesic action but no respiratory depression or after-effects, allowing the patient to be comfortable yet accessible and able to change position during the procedure, but then to recover rapidly afterwards. The nearest approach to this ideal is currently given by IV delivery, through an in-dwelling plastic cannula, of a benzodiazepine hypnotic such as midazolam (1–3 mg) either given alone or combined with a low dose of an opiate such as fentanyl (50–100 μg). The benzodiazepine produces anxiolytic, sedational, and amnesic effects while the opiate contributes analgesia and slight euphoria. Midazolam can cause significant amnesia, so much so that the patient may remember nothing of the procedure or discussion of the findings immediately afterwards. This should be borne in mind before patient discharge as a repeat discussion with the clinical team is often required.

In general, only a small dose of benzodiazepine should be given unless the patient is very anxious. The initial injection is given slowly over a period of at least 1 minute, "titrating" the dose to some extent by observing the patient's conscious state and ability to talk coherently—some patients merely become loquacious. A small initial "starter dose" makes it possible to judge during initial insertion through the sigmoid whether the rest of the procedure is likely to be easy or difficult, and whether the patient is pain-sensitive or not. A lower dosage is used for older, sicker patients but the amount required is unpredictable; younger patients may tolerate maximal doses and remain (fairly) coherent. If in doubt it is safer to underestimate the titration and give more later if necessary.

Use extra opiate rather than more benzodiazepine if extra medication is needed. Benzodiazepines make some patients even more restless and have no painkilling properties. Benzodiazepines and opiates potentiate each other, not only in effectiveness but also in side effects such as depression of respiration and blood pressure. Pulse oximetry should, therefore, be routinely used with low dose (2 L/min) nasal oxygen in all sedated patients—with the caveat that this is contraindicated in severe chronic obstructive airways disease, where CO_2 capnography would ideally be used.

Deep sedation and anesthesia

Propofol (Diprivan®), a short-lived IV emulsion anesthetic agent, is widely used for colonoscopy in some countries (United States, France, Germany, Australia) and increasingly in others. It should ideally be administered by an anesthetist because of the significant risk of marked respiratory depression but, with appropriate training and safeguards, has been extensively employed by endoscopists with an anesthetic-trained nurse assistant, with apparent safety and satisfactory results. Its short duration of action—giving full recovery within about 30 minutes—is an advantage over excessive doses of conventional sedatives. However, the patient can be rendered insensible and unable to cooperate with changes of position or to give early warning of excessive pain. With experience, anesthesiologists learn a light-touch approach, using small doses of propofol to protect the patient during potentially uncomfortable moments such as passage around the mid-sigmoid or sigmoid/descending junction. Once the scope is straight, very little sedation is required and frequently none at all for the scope withdrawal, which is often the longest part of the procedure. With this approach, and the very short half-life of the drug, the patient is often completely recovered by the end of the procedure, can receive the results without subsequent amnesia, and is ready to leave the department within 30 minutes.

General anesthesia may be required in select cases where, for example, conventional or deep sedation has failed due to procedure tolerance or where a prolonged procedure is expected (e.g. complex polypectomy). These patients require careful pre-assessment and those with significant risk factors should be reviewed by an anesthetist.

Antagonists

The availability of antagonists to benzodiazepines (flumazenil) and opiates (naloxone) is invaluable, providing a safety measure for the rare occasions when inadvertent oversedation has occurred. These drugs should never be used routinely to reverse oversedated patients, a dangerous and outdated practice. There is no reversal agent for propofol so if transient oversedation occurs, the airway must be managed with bag and mask ventilation, waiting 1–2 minutes until the propofol has been metabolized.

Antispasmodics

Antispasmodics induce colonic relaxation for at least 5–10 minutes and help to optimize the view during examination of a hypercontractile colon. Either hyoscine *N*-butylbromide (Buscopan®) 10–20 mg IV (in countries where it can be prescribed) or glucagon 0.5–1 mg IV are effective. Fears about anticholinergics initiating glaucoma are misplaced because patients previously diagnosed are completely protected by their eye drops, and those with undiagnosed chronic glaucoma are best served by precipitating an acute attack, which will cause the diagnosis to be made. Patients should be told to seek medical attention if they experience any eye pain. Glucagon is more expensive but has no ocular or prostatic side effects. Buscopan does cause a transient tachycardia and, therefore, caution is required in patients with ischemic heart disease or known cardiac arrythmias.

Intravenous antispasmodics have a relatively short duration of action, leading some endoscopists to give them only when the colonoscope is fully inserted. Experienced endoscopists, sure of a rapid procedure, may give them at the start. There is an unproven suspicion that the bowel is rendered more redundant and atonic by antispasmodics and will be more difficult to examine; on the contrary, we find that the view is improved and colonoscope insertion is faster after using antispasmodics, particularly if there is sigmoid colon diverticulosis or the scope tip diameter is slightly increased by the use of a cuff or cap. Benzodiazepines have a weak antispasmodic effect, relaxing most colons except for those that are "irritable" or spastic. In the unsedated patient, therefore, antispasmodics may be particularly helpful, and the anti-muscarinic effects can also protect against vasovagal episodes in patients who are prone to this.

Equipment—present and future

This chapter aims to "make colonoscopy easy," but this also depends to a fair degree on the instrumentation used. We have tried to generalize and be noncommercial in approach, as the colonoscopes of all manufacturers are serviceable and we have used many of them—although with individual preferences. A number of ingenious innovations are under current evaluation, designed to propel or guide the colonoscope or to view the colon more easily. While enthusiastic for future improvements and innovations, we have deliberately excluded these from the present account, which describes the best ways to manage the "push" colonoscopes currently used, including those with in-built stiffening or "magnetic imaging" facilities.

Colonoscopes

Colonoscopes are engineered similarly to upper gastrointestinal endoscopes, but are longer, have a wider diameter (for better twist or torque control), and have a more flexible shaft. The bending section of the colonoscope tip is longer and more gently curved, avoiding impaction in acute bends such as the splenic flexure. Ideal future colonoscopes ought to have electronic steering to make single-handed insertion easier; present angulation control mechanisms are almost unchanged from those of early gastrocameras and gastroscopes and are poorly suited to the more finicky steering movements during colonoscopy.

The introduction of variable stiffness instruments avoids the need to choose the "right colonoscope for the job" at the stage of purchase or before starting examination of a particular patient—especially one known or predicted to have a long "difficult" colon or severe adhesions (see also "Variable-stiffness colonoscopes" below). Long colonoscopes (165–180 cm) are able to reach the cecum even in redundant colons and so are our preferred routine choice of instrument. Intermediate-length instruments (130–140 cm) are considered by some, including most German or Japanese endoscopists, to be a good compromise, almost always reaching the cecum. The only advantage of using 70 cm flexible sigmoidoscopes for limited examinations is that the endoscopist knows from the onset that the procedure will be limited, thus avoiding the temptation to go further. However, as flexible sigmoidoscopy can be performed with a longer instrument (a pediatric colonoscope is ideal); there is no reason to purchase flexible sigmoidoscopes for an endoscopy unit, although they may have an essential role in the office of a primary-care physician or an outpatient facility.

Variable-stiffness colonoscopes

Variable-stiffness colonoscopes (Innoflex®, Olympus Corporation) have a twist control on the shaft (Fig 7.2a) that forcibly compresses and rigidifies an internal steel coil similar to that in a bicycle brake cable (Fig 7.2b,c and Video 7.2). Compressing the coil stiffens it and the shaft/insertion tube within which it lies. The distal 30 cm to the tip of the bending section is left "floppy" and easily deflectable at all times. The bonus of using a variable-stiffness colonoscope is that, without having to withdraw and exchange instruments, the endoscopist can select a relatively "floppy" shaft mode to pass looping sections of the colon, then twist to apply "stiff" mode, so discouraging re-looping after the scope has been straightened out, typically at the splenic flexure.

Variable-stiffness scopes thus combine, in one colonoscope, many of the virtues of both standard and pediatric instruments. They prove significantly easier and less traumatic to use in most patients found previously to be "difficult" to examine—especially where the problem was due to uncontrollable looping and discomfort. As any first-time colonoscopy may prove to be difficult, a long, variable-stiffness instrument is our "colonoscope of choice."

Pediatric colonoscopes

Pediatric colonoscopes of small diameter (9–12 mm) are available with either standard, "floppy," or variable-stiffness characteristics. They are invaluable for the examination of infants and children up to 2–3 years of age but also have a role to play in older children and adult endoscopy and are the preferred choice of some skilled endoscopists. As well as allowing examination of strictures, anastomoses, or stomas that would be impassable with the full-sized colonoscope, they are often much easier to pass through areas of tethered postoperative adhesions or severe diverticular disease. The pediatric colonoscope bending section is more flexible, making it easier to obtain a retroverted view of some awkwardly placed polyps, whether in the distal or proximal colon, in order to ensure complete removal. Floppy pediatric instruments are also particularly comfortable and easy to insert to the splenic flexure, tending to conform to the colon in a spontaneous spiral configuration, which avoids difficulty in passing to the descending colon.

For limited adult examinations, as for strictures or diverticular disease, a gastroscope can also be used (it has the bonus of an even shorter bending section, but the disadvantage of limited downward angling capability). The stiff shaft of a gastroscope, however, makes it less suitable than the pediatric colonoscope for examinations of small children and babies.

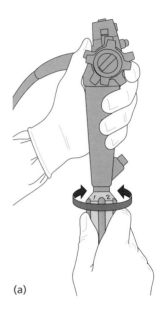
(a)

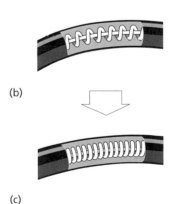
(b)

(c)

Fig 7.2 (a) Variable-stiffness colonoscopes have a twist control on the shaft. (b) A pull-wire within an internal spring-steel coil (c) compresses the coil and stiffens it (and the scope).

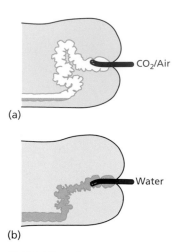

(a)

(b)

Fig 7.3 Effect of using (a) gas or (b) water for colonoscope insertion in left lateral position.

Water-assisted insertion

A major recent change in insertion technique has been brought about by the introduction of commercially available water pumps allied to an additional small water-jet channel built into modern scopes and controlled via a foot pedal (use the nondominant foot to control the water pump, which leaves the dominant foot free to control electrosurgical unit pedals if needed; Fig 7.5 and Video 7.3). The combination allows a water jet for irrigation, cleaning, and infusion of water during insertion. Most colonoscopists have now adopted a water-assisted insertion technique whereby water is used to open up and gently distend the colon to find the lumen. CO_2 insufflation is minimized to keep the colon collapsed around the scope and air pockets are aspirated prior to deeper insertion. There are two main variations of water insertion. The first, called *water exchange*, involves water irrigation and aspiration of fluid prior to scope advancement (gas insufflation not used) and the second, *water immersion*, involves progressive insertion with water irrigation (gas insufflation can be used) and aspiration of water primarily during withdrawal. In fact, in our experience, a *hybrid technique* is optimal, whereby the left colon is intubated predominately with water to the splenic flexure, with CO_2 used only if required (e.g. poor bowel preparation), then low-volume CO_2 predominately used from splenic flexure to the cecum. The advantage of water, particularly in the left colon, is that it weighs down the colon, keeps it collapsed and reduces looping, thereby causing less stretch and discomfort and enabling nearly straight passage of the scope from the sigmoid to the descending colon in around 50% of patients (Fig 7.3). Use of CO_2 insufflation from the splenic flexure to the cecum generally proves quicker than using water alone, without causing undue distention or patient discomfort.

Gas insufflation: Air or carbon dioxide?

CO_2 insufflation is now widely used and has many benefits compared to room air. CO_2 was originally used instead of air because of the explosive potential of colonic gases during electrosurgery. However, with the exception of bowel preparation using mannitol, a thing of the past, the prepared colon has been shown to have no residual explosive gas. Even for routine examinations, the use of CO_2 offers the striking advantage that it is cleared from the colon 100 times faster than air (through the circulation, to the lungs, and then breathed out). This means that 10–15 minutes after finishing an exam using CO_2 insufflation, the colon and small intestine are free of any gas and the patient's abdomen is deflated. In contrast, air distension can remain and cause abdominal bloating and discomfort for many hours post-procedure, which is particularly distressing for patients with irritable bowel syndrome. In the unlikely event of perforation or gas leak (pneumoperitoneum), air under pressure would add to the hazard, whereas rapidly absorbed CO_2 and a well-prepared colon would markedly reduce it. Patients with ileus, pseudo-obstruction, stricturing, severe colitis, diverticular disease, or functional bowel disorder particularly benefit from the added safety and comfort of using CO_2 rather than air insufflation.

Low-pressure, controlled-flow CO_2 delivery systems with fail-safe pressure-reducing features are available commercially. These remove any risk of the patient being exposed to the hazard of high pressure from the cylinder in the event of failure of the conventional flow-meter. A CO_2 insufflation valve can be substituted for the usual air/water valve, but in practice it is easier to connect the CO_2 supply to the water bottle (Fig 7.4) and use the normal air/water valve, as the modest leakage of CO_2 into room atmosphere is of no more consequence than having another person in the room.

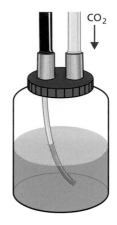

Fig 7.4 Connect the CO_2 supply directly to the water bottle.

Instrument checks and troubleshooting

The functionality of the colonoscope should be checked before examination, because imperfections can be difficult to spot or tedious to remedy during it. Colonoscopy can be difficult enough without adding problems in instrument performance.

Insufflation/lens washing checks are essential before every colonoscopy. Because CO_2/air flow and water wash share a short common exit channel (Fig 3.5), the quickest way of simultaneously checking air/water functionality is to depress the water-wash valve and look for a healthy squirt from the scope tip. Once the procedure has started it is difficult to assess inadequacy of CO_2/air flow and insufflation pressure, the resulting poor view making it seem that the colonoscopy is "difficult" or the colon apparently "hypercontractile." A great deal of wasted time can be avoided by noticing any such problem before starting, and correcting it or changing instruments.

If there is no insufflation at all, check the light source. Is the CO_2/air pump switched on? Are the umbilical and water-bottle connections pushed in fully and the water bottle screwed on? Is the rubber O-ring in place on the water-bottle connection? Is the air/water valve in good condition and seated properly (or the CO_2 valve in position where relevant), as it will otherwise allow air leakage? If in doubt, proper CO_2/air insufflation pressure and flow can be proven by blowing up a rubber glove wound over the scope tip.

Water-wash failure is unusual, except because of an empty water bottle or a faulty air/water valve.

Suction failure can be caused by valve blockage, which should be obvious on careful inspection or changing the valve, or by debris blocking the suction channel. If this is in the shaft it can be dislodged by water-syringing through the biopsy port. Removing the suction valve and covering the opening on the control head with a finger is a quick way of improving suction pressure and can result in rapid clearance of the whole system (as when sucking polyp specimens). Applying the sucker tube directly to the suction channel opening can also be effective in clearing particulate debris. As a final resort the whole suction system can be cleared by retrograde-syringing using a 50-mL bladder syringe and tubing attached to the suction port on the umbilical. Push the suction valve and also cover the biopsy port during this procedure to avoid unpleasant (refluxed) surprises.

Water pump: always check that the water pump is producing a vigorous flow of water from the scope tip on pressing the foot pedal. If there is a reduced water pressure, then there may be an air lock in the compression tubing of the pump or, alternatively, the connecting tubing has been incorrectly set up or the sterile water bottle may be empty and needs replacing.

Ergonomics

The room should be set up with ergonomics in mind to allow maintenance of a neutral body posture with the least possible muscle strain (e.g. adjusting bed height, monitor, and electrosurgical unit position).

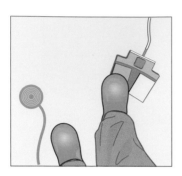

Fig 7.5 Positioning of foot pedals for electrosurgical unit and water pump. The dominant foot is used to control the electrosurgical unit.

• *Monitor:* position directly in front of the endoscopist with the center of the screen at resting eye position (15 to 25 degrees below the horizon) to help prevent neck strain.

• *Bed:* adjust to a height between 0 and 10 cm below the elbow height to allow a good working range of movement of both forearms.

• *Endoscopic processor:* locate behind the endoscopist and in line with the patient's anorectum.

• *Electrosurgical unit:* position opposite endoscopist so settings can easily be checked prior to therapy.

• *Foot pedals* for all devices should be placed in a comfortable position to avoid twisting or looking down during the procedure (Fig 7.5).

• *Nurse assistants* need free access to accessories, drugs and a specimen processing area.

• *Trainers* should position themselves at the foot of the bed alongside the trainee to maximize views of the patient, monitor, and trainee's hands.

Accessories and attachments

All the usual accessories are used through the working channel of the colonoscope, including biopsy forceps, snares, retrieval forceps or nets, injection needles, spray catheters, dilating balloons, etc. Long and intermediate-length accessories work equally well down shorter instruments, so it is sensible to order all accessories to suit the longest instrument in routine use. Other manufacturers' accessories also work down any particular instrument and, as some are better than others, it is worth taking advice from colleagues when buying replacements.

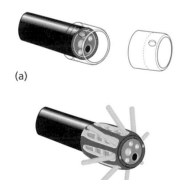

(a)

(b)

Fig 7.6 Scope tip attachments: (a) cap; (b) cuff.

Tip-mounted scope attachments, such as a cap or cuff, can be added to the scope tip prior to colonoscope insertion (Fig 7.6):

• *Cap-assisted colonoscopy* uses a clear plastic cap attached to the tip of the colonoscope to keep the mucosa away from the lens when negotiating tight bends and can improve mucosal visualization on withdrawal. It is also valuable for therapeutic procedures in cases of complex polypectomy.

• *Cuff-assisted colonoscopy* uses a device with flexible arms attached to the colonoscope tip to help flatten folds to optimize both mucosal and overall views. This has been shown to improve polyp detection rate.

Magnetic imaging of endoscope loops

It helps to know what shaft loops have formed during colonoscope insertion and where the tip is. In 1993 two UK groups introduced prototype magnetic imagers to "position-sense" the configuration of the instrument shaft, producing a moving 3D image on a computer monitor. Small coils within the instrument (or in a probe passed down its instrumentation channel) generate pulsed magnetic fields that energize larger sensor coils in a dish alongside the patient, computed to produce a real-time monitor graphic display (Fig 7.7). Three systems are now commercially available from the three major endoscope manufacturers which use coils incorporated within the shaft of the scope. The ScopeGuide® system from Olympus is demonstrated in Video 7.4. These produce fields no stronger than those of a television set and are safe for continuous use, except for patients with cardiac pacemakers.

In use, magnetic imaging makes many previously difficult and looping colons much quicker and easier to intubate, and also ensures that the endoscopist knows at all times where the colonoscope tip has reached and what loops have formed. It rationalizes many of the uncertainties of colonoscopy, and can be a boon to both beginners and experts. The magnetic imager is particularly helpful in patients with a long colon, who can be preselected on the basis of a history of constipation or the presence of hemorrhoids, or if they report a delayed response to bowel preparation.

Anatomy

Embryological anatomy (and "difficult colonoscopy")

The embryology of colon development is complex and somewhat unpredictable, especially in terms of its outcome for mesenteries and fixations, which probably explains the extraordinarily variable configurations into which the colon can be pushed during colonoscopy (Video 7.5). The fetal intestine and colon initially develop as a functionless muscle tube joined at its midpoint to the yolk stalk. This muscle tube lengthens into a U-shape on a longitudinal mesentery (Fig 7.8a). As the embryo at this 5-week stage is only 1 cm long, the lengthening intestine and colon (Fig 7.8b) are forced out into the umbilical hernia (Fig 7.8c). The gut loop thus differentiates

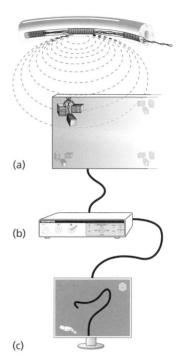

(a)

(b)

(c)

Fig 7.7 (a) Small coils within the scope generate magnetic fields, (b) energizing larger coils in the receiver dish beside the patient; (c) the signals are then processed as a 3D image on the monitor.

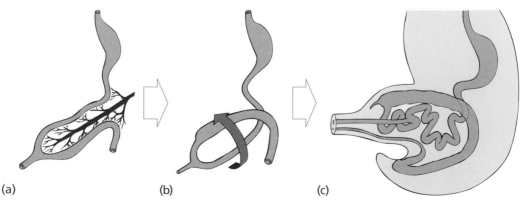

(a)   (b)   (c)

Fig 7.8 (a) The fetal intestine and colon start on a longitudinal mesentery, (b) then rotate as the small intestine elongates, (c) and from 5 weeks (1 cm embryo) to 10 weeks (4 cm embryo) are in the umbilical hernia.

into the small and large intestine outside the abdominal cavity. By the third month of development the embryo is 4 cm long and there is room within the peritoneal cavity for first the small, and then the large, intestine to be returned into the abdomen. This occurs in a fairly predictable manner, with the end result being that the colon is rotated around so that the cecum lies in the right hypochondrium and the descending colon is to the left of the abdomen (Fig 7.9a).

With further elongation of the colon, the cecum normally migrates down to the right iliac fossa. At this stage, the mesentery of the transverse colon is free but the mesenteries of the descending and ascending colon, pushed against the peritoneum of the posterior abdominal wall by the fluid-filled and bulky small intestine, fuse with it so that the ascending and descending colon typically becomes retroperitoneal and fixed (although not always; Fig 7.9b).

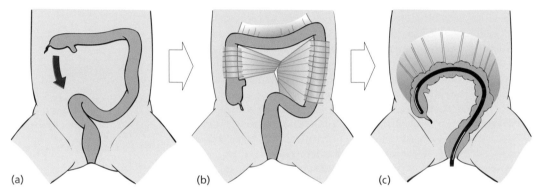

(a)   (b)   (c)

Fig 7.9 (a) The embryonic colon extends on its mesentery, (b) then partial fusion of the mesentery and peritoneum occurs at 3 months, (c) although sometimes the colon remains mobile.

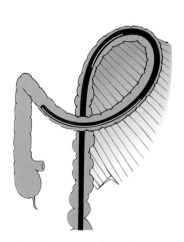

Fig 7.10 Persistent descending mesocolon or mesentery.

Incomplete fusion of the mesocolon to the posterior wall of the abdomen results in a relatively free-floating colon. Such a mobile colon can be a nightmare for the colonoscopist, because there are no fixed points at which to obtain leverage, and few of the usual "tricks of the trade" will work, as most of them depend on withdrawal and leverage against fixations. The explanation for this variation from normal development may be the failure of enteric innervation of the intestinal muscle tube in early embryonic development. An atonic, bulky, and dysfunctional fetal intestine and colon will be retained longer than usual outside the abdomen in the umbilical hernia, until the developing abdominal cavity is large enough to re-accommodate it. Delayed return of a large colon into the abdomen will cause it to miss the "milestone moment" for retroperitoneal fixation and fusion to occur (usually by 10–12 weeks after conception). The long, mobile (and increasingly dysfunctional) colon may present clinically in childhood with straining at stool and bleeding, in teenage years with constipation, or in adulthood with hemorrhoids, variable bowel habit, and flatulence.

Endoscopically such a colon is noted to be unusually capacious, long, and often atypically looping, but it can also be dramatically squashed down and shortened when the colonoscope is withdrawn at the cecum (typically to a length of only 50–60 cm), proving the lack of fixations. Suggestive evidence that this is a genetically determined abnormality of development is the frequency of other first-degree relatives (especially on the female side and sometimes over several generations) known to have disturbance of habit, constipation, or flatulence. If endoscoped or imaged, the colon of such relatives (also their stomach and small intestine) are found to be similarly large, long, and mobile.

How often such failure of fusion, persistent colonic mesentery, and mobility occurs is not clear from the literature. A persistent descending mesocolon has been found at postmortem in 36% with an ascending mesocolon in 10%. The persistence of a descending mesocolon explains most of the excessive loops and strange configurations that can be caused by the colonoscope passing the left colon and splenic flexure (Fig 7.10). Occasionally the cecum fails to descend and becomes fixed in the right hypochondrium (Fig 7.11); in others, where a free mesocolon persists, the cecum is mobile and can be pushed into weird configurations by the endoscope (Fig 7.12).

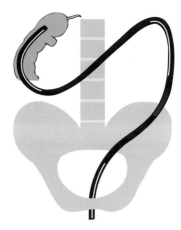

Fig 7.11 Inverted cecum.

3-D adult colon configuration

The in-utero colon, originally the distal part of a floppy mid-line tube, has, when fully-developed, variable segments of retroperitoneal fixation or mesenteric mobility. These anatomic variables have consequences for the endoscopist that can potentially be helpful. The conventional image of colon configuration typically shows an unnaturally short sigmoid colon, whereas the sigmoid is long and free-floating on its "mesocolon"—so it can be collapsed down, distended with gas, or stretched up by instrument pressure (Fig 7.13).

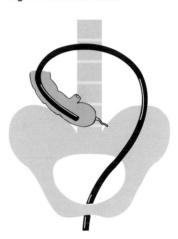

Fig 7.12 Mobile cecum.

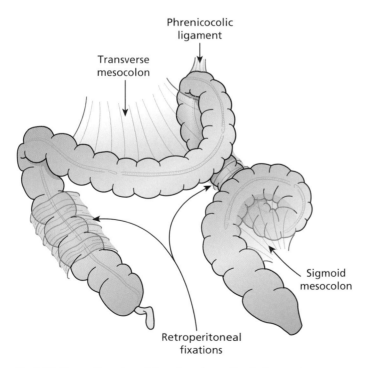

Phrenicocolic
ligament

Transverse
mesocolon

Sigmoid
mesocolon

Retroperitoneal
fixations

Fig 7.13 The configuration of the colon when inflated, showing its attachments and fixations.

For convenience of insertion most patients are examined starting in the left lateral position, with gravitational effects on the mobile sigmoid, transverse colon, and flexures. Fluid will flow toward the descending colon and gas will preferentially rise to distend the distal sigmoid and proximal colon. Patient position change to supine or right lateral position will reverse these effects and affect the configuration of the flexures proximally. Dynamic position change during colonoscopy can be used to aid insertion and improve visualization (Fig 7.14), assuming that the patient has not been oversedated and can cooperate with the transfer. Because the configuration of the colon is variable, Fig 7.14 is a guide to the most commonly used positions at specific anatomical points during insertion, but sometimes different positions are required, and a trial-and-error process must occur to find the position that gives optimal visualization.

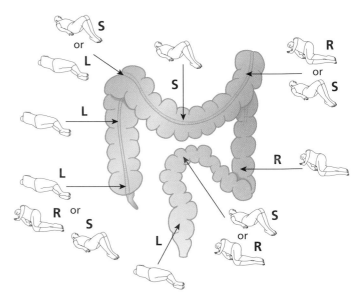

Fig 7.14 Dynamic position changes to facilitate insertion of the colonoscope (L: left lateral, R: right lateral, S: supine).

Changing a patient's position does take a few seconds to achieve, and movement can be cumbersome if the patient is obese, has impaired mobility, or is oversedated. We, therefore, change position if "stuck" despite attempting direct passage using the approaches suggested later in this chapter.

Making a position change to right or left lateral can be made into a simple routine (Video 7.6):

1 change hands, to hold the instrument control body in the right hand;

2 use your left hand to help the patient raise their legs slightly;

3 slide the shaft through to the other side of the legs;

4 the patient can then turn over.

Providing the shaft is kept away from the patient's heels there is nothing to go wrong. The whole position-change maneuver takes at most 20–30 seconds in a lightly sedated patient. Subsequent position changes take less time still, because the patient understands what is required.

Endoscopic anatomy

The *anal canal*, 3 cm long, extends up to the squamocolumnar junction or "dentate line." Sensory innervation, and hence mucosal pain sensation, may in some subjects extend up to 5–7 cm into the distal rectum. Around the canal are the anal sphincters, normally in tonic contraction. The anus may be deformed, scarred, or made sensitive by present or previous local pathology, including hemorrhoids or other conditions. Normal subjects may also be sore from the effects of bowel preparation.

There are three potentially serious consequences from the fact that the hemorrhoidal veins drain into the systemic (not the portal) circulation:

1 Mistakenly snaring a "pile" can result in catastrophic hemorrhage.

2 Injecting intramucosal epinephrine (adrenaline) at a concentration over 1:200,000 before sessile polypectomy in the distal rectum has a serious risk of inducing potentially fatal cardiac or circulatory events (whereas the colonic vasculature drains via the portal system, so the liver metabolizes the higher concentrations of epinephrine often used proximally).

3 Therapy may translocate bacteria directly into the systemic circulation, so we generally give a broad-spectrum antibiotic such as co-amoxiclav to cover more invasive low rectal procedures.

The *rectum*, reaching 15 cm proximal to the anal verge, may have a capacious "ampulla" in its mid-part as well as three or more prominent partial or "semilunar" folds (valves of Houston) that create potential blind spots, in any of which (as well as the distal rectum) the endoscopist can miss significant pathology. Digital examination, direct inspection, and, where appropriate, a rigid rectoscope/proctoscope are needed for complete examination of the area. "Video-proctoscopy" (see "Video-proctoscopy/anoscopy" below) is a convenient way of visualizing the anal canal, rectal mucosal prolapse, or hemorrhoids, but not the remainder of the rectum (which requires inflation for careful inspection and, where possible, instrument retroversion). Prominent, somewhat tortuous, veins are a normal feature of the rectal mucosa and should not be confused with the rare, markedly serpiginous veins of a hemangioma or the distended, tortuous varices seen in some cases of portal hypertension.

The rectum is extraperitoneal for its distal 10–12 cm, making this part relatively safe for therapeutic maneuvers, but proximally it enters the abdominal cavity, invested in peritoneum. When invasive procedures such as endoscopic mucosal resection (EMR) or endoscopic submucosal resection (ESD) are performed, special attention should be made to avoid perforation, particularly anteriorly in female patients where a long pouch of Douglas may make the intraperitoneal part of the rectal wall lower than anticipated. Whereas the colon surface is devoid of sensory nerves and pain-free, patients may experience "burning pain" for up to 5–7 cm

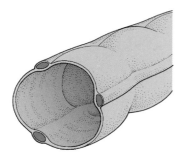

Fig 7.15 The longitudinal muscle bundles (teniae coli) can bulge visibly into the colon.

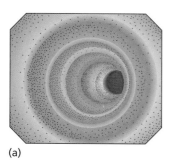

(a)

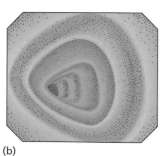

(b)

Fig 7.16 (a) The distal colon appearance is usually circular, whereas (b) the transverse colon is usually triangular.

above the anal verge. This is easily managed for polypectomy by intramucosal local anesthetic injection (1% lidocaine added to the submucosal lifting solution).

Mucosal "microanatomy" is visible to the discerning endoscopist, particularly with the emergence of high-resolution and high-magnification colonoscopes. This includes the shiny surface coating of mucus, around 30% of the mucosal cells being mucus-secreting and described as "goblet cells" because of their flask-shaped mucus-containing inclusions. The "highlights" reflected off the surface by the protective mucus layer can show up fine underlying detail, such as the arc impressions of circular muscle fibers or the dappled, sieve-like reflections caused by the microscopic crypt or pit openings. Minor abnormalities, such as prominent lymphoid follicles and the smallest polyps or flat adenomas, often first catch the endoscopist's eye through such reflections or "light reflexes" off the mucus layer. The mucosal columnar epithelium, around 50 cells thick, is transparent (unlike the horny squamous epithelium of the skin surface) and through it can be seen, often in exquisite detail, the paired venules and arterioles that make up the normal submucosal "vessel pattern."

Colonic musculature develops into three external longitudinal muscle bundles, or teniae coli, and within these, the wrapping of circular muscle fibers. Both muscle layers are sometimes visible to the endoscopist (Fig 7.15). One or more of the teniae may be seen endoscopically as a longitudinal fold, because an unusually thin-walled, capacious colon can bulge out between its teniae. The circular musculature is seen as fine reflective corrugations under the mucosal surface, particularly in "spastic" or hypertonic colons. The distal colon, needing to cope with formed stools, has markedly thicker circular musculature than in the proximal colon, resulting in a tubular appearance (Fig 7.16a) broken by the ridged indentations of the haustral folds. The thinner-walled transverse colon is kept in triangular shape by the three teniae (Fig 7.16b).

Haustral folds segment the interior of the colon. Those that are prominent in the proximal colon sometimes create "blind spots," whereas they can be hypertrophied in sigmoid diverticular disease, also creating mechanical difficulties for the endoscopist.

In elderly subjects the sigmoid colon anatomy is often narrowed and deformed internally by the thickened circular muscle rings of hypertrophic diverticular disease, and sometimes also fixed externally by pericolic post-inflammatory processes or adhesions. Redundant and prolapsing mucosal folds overlying the muscular rings in diverticular disease may appear reddened from traumatization, and sometimes show focal inflammation histologically as well.

External structures can be seen through the colonic wall, typically as the blue-gray discoloration of the spleen or the liver proximally. Vascular pulsations of the adjacent left iliac artery are often visible in the sigmoid, and right iliac artery pulsations are occasionally visible proximally. Marked aortic or cardiac pulsation can be seen in the transverse colon. Small intestinal gas distension or peristaltic activity may occasionally be visible through the colon wall, especially when it indents the cecal pole.

Insertion

Pre-procedure checks should be made on all functions of the endoscope, light source, and accessories before insertion (see "Instrument checks and troubleshooting" above). A clean lens is also important.

Insertion through the anus should be gentle. The instrument tip is unavoidably blunt (the lenses mean that it cannot be streamlined) so too fast or forcible insertion may be painful for patients with tight sphincters or a sore anal region. The squamous epithelium of the anus and the sensory mechanisms of the anal sphincters are the most pain-sensitive areas in the colorectum.

There are several ways of inserting the scope (Video 7.7):

• *Start with two gloves* on the right hand and perform a digital rectal examination with a generous amount of lubricant before inserting the instrument, both to check for pathology in this potentially "blind" area and to prelubricate and relax the anal canal. The instrument tip is passed in by pressing obliquely, supported by the examiner's forefinger until the sphincter relaxes (Fig 7.17a).

• *Use the thumb to push the tip in* along the examining forefinger as this withdraws from the anal canal (Fig 7.17b). The tendency of the bending section to flex can be avoided by starting with it straight, fixing the angulation control brakes and pressing in gently.

• *In the "direct" approach*, a large blob of lubricant jelly is spread over the anal orifice and the instrument is inserted directly through it (Fig 7.17c), which saves a glove and a few seconds. However, a digital rectal examination must have been performed before direct insertion. Inflating CO_2/air down the endoscope while pressing the tip into the anal canal gives direct vision and facilitates insertion.

Tight or tonic sphincters may take time to relax; asking the patient to "bear down" is said to help this. Allowing an extra 15–20 seconds for sphincter relaxation can be a humane start to proceedings, especially for a patient with anorectal pathology or anismus. The sphincters of colitis patients are noticeably more tonic than normal, presumably because of the long-standing need to keep control and avoid leakage.

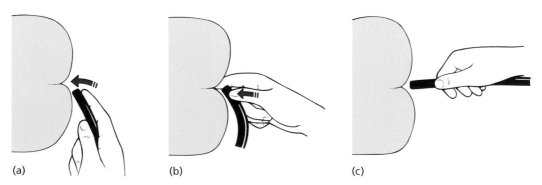

(a) (b) (c)

Fig 7.17 Different methods of colonoscope insertion: (a) finger support of the bending section; (b) the tip pushed in as the examining finger withdraws; or (c) straight on through the jelly.

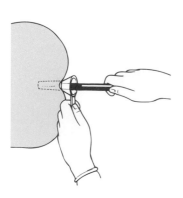

Fig 7.18 Video-proctoscopy (anoscopy).

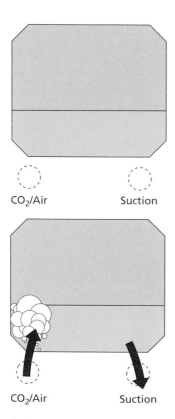

CO_2/Air   Suction

CO_2/Air   Suction

Fig 7.19 The colonoscope suction/instrumentation port opens below and to the right of the view (5 o'clock); the CO_2/air port below and to the left (7 o'clock).

Video-proctoscopy/anoscopy

Rigid proctoscopy has an important role in selected patients with bleeding after "normal colonoscopy" to inspect the anorectal area for mucosal prolapse, hemorrhoids, or other pathology. The patient can also be shown the anal canal or hemorrhoidal appearances by the simple expedient of inserting the video endoscope tip up the proctoscope once its insertion trocar is removed (the rectum will deflate and is poorly seen). The colonoscope simultaneously provides a convenient source of illumination and an excellent way of showing the patient any skin tags, anal papillae, or other local features that they could not normally see. The endoscopist performs this *video-proctoscopy or anoscopy* (Fig 7.18) from the monitor view, with the opportunity for taking a videotaped or printed record. In many cases of "unexplained bleeding" this will convincingly show the patient the likely (hemorrhoidal or mucosal) traumatic source of the problem.

Rectal insertion

A "red-out" is often the first view after the scope has been inserted into the rectum. This is because the lens is pressed against the rectal mucosa. The following steps should be performed, in sequence (Video 7.7).

1 *Irrigate* water to slightly distend the rectum and perform water exchange to provide a clean underwater view. Often there is some retained residue in the rectum and exchange of cloudy fluid for clear water is required to be able to see the direction of the lumen underwater. If irrigation is unavailable, *insufflate a small amount of CO_2/air* to find the direction of the rectal lumen.

2 *Pull back and angulate* or rotate slightly to find the lumen. This is the first of many times during the examination when withdrawal, inspection, (and cerebration) bring success more quickly than pushing blindly.

3 *When suctioning or exchanging fluid, rotate the view* so that fluid lies inferiorly at the 6 o'clock position. The suction port of the colonoscope tip lies just below the bottom right-hand corner of the image (Fig 7.19) and should be selectively placed in fluid before activating the suction valve. Coordination will be required between shaft rotation (with the right hand) and synchronous up or down angulation (with the left hand) so as to keep the view. During the examination phase of colonoscopy, *a skilled single-handed endoscopist often uses twist to torque-steer or "corkscrew" the tip*. The capacious rectum is the ideal place in which to practice this, as the shaft is inevitably straight, and no force should be needed for precise finger-control.

4 *Aspirate excess fluid, residue*, and any gas pockets to shorten and collapse the rectum. The warm, lubricated colonoscope shaft moving in and out often gives the patient a distressing illusion of being incontinent. Knowing that there is no excess rectal fluid to leak out, and that any gas can be passed without fear of an accident, is a bonus for everyone (not least the endoscopist).

5 *Push in*, finally, but only when an adequate view has been obtained, and only as fast as a reasonable view can be obtained.

6 *Torque-steer round* the first few bends, using up or down angulation and shaft-twist alone to achieve most lateral movements, rather than unnecessarily using the lateral (left/right) angulation control knob. Torque-steering (with controlled shaft-twisting or corkscrewing movements) is an essential part of skilled colonoscopy.

Retroversion

Retroversion, being mildly uncomfortable, is usually performed just before scope withdrawal at the end of the procedure. It is important because, although the rectum is relatively capacious, it can be surprisingly difficult to examine it completely, even with a wide-angle lens. Care is needed to combine angulating and twisting movements sufficiently to see behind the major folds, or valves of Houston. In a capacious rectum the most distal part is a potential blind spot, but the generous size of such a large rectal ampulla will usually make tip retroflexion relatively easy. To perform it:

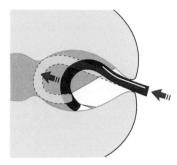

Fig 7.20 Angulate both controls, twist and *push in* to retrovert in the rectum.

1 *pull back to the widest part of the distal rectum*
2 *angulate both controls fully*
3 *twist the shaft vigorously and simultaneously*
4 *push inward to invert the tip toward the anal verge* (Fig 7.20).

   Retroversion is not always possible in a small or narrowed rectum, but when this is the case the wide-angled (170°, nearly "fish-eye") lens of the endoscope should see everything with minimal risk of blind spots.

Handling "single-handed," "two-handed," or two-person?

Most skilled endoscopists favor the one-person "single-handed" approach, in which the colonoscopist manages the angulation controls and valves with one hand and inserts or twists the shaft with the other (Video 7.7). However, there are many who use two hands on the angulation controls and a few experts who work successfully with the "two-person" method, using an assistant to manipulate the shaft.

Two-person colonoscopy

Two-person colonoscopy relies on an assistant to handle the shaft while the endoscopist uses both hands to manage the control body of the instrument, with the left hand working the up/down angulation control knob and air/water/suction valves but the right hand adjusting the right/left angulation control knob. Colonoscope control ergonomics are based on those of gastroscopes (and originally gastrocameras) and so are fundamentally designed for "two-handed" steering. However, whereas the short and stiff insertion tube of a gastroscope is easy for the endoscopist to control, the long and floppy shaft of a colonoscope is not. In this approach the assistant, therefore, performs the role delegated to the right hand of the single-handed endoscopist, pushing and pulling according to the spoken instructions of the endoscopist. A good assistant learns to feel the shaft to some extent and may apply some twist. More often, however, the assistant pushes with concealed gusto and causes unnecessary loops that are not apparent to the endoscopist but painful for the patient.

Unless endoscopist/assistant teamwork is skilled and interactive, the two-person approach to colonoscopy can be as illogical and clumsy as would be expected of two people attempting any other intricate task, neither quite knowing what the other is doing.

In occasional difficult situations, for instance when passing an awkward angulation or snaring a difficult polyp, any endoscopist may justifiably involve the assistant briefly to steady or control the shaft. Otherwise, for the generality of colonoscopy, we do not recommend the two-person handling approach.

"Two-handed" one-person technique

The "two-handed technique" is a common compromise approach, the endoscopist using both hands on the angulation controls when required, but also handling the shaft for insertion and torque control. The two-handed approach is mainly used by those with small hands, who find it difficult to activate the lateral (left/right) angulation control knob except by use of the right hand. Each time a lateral angulation is made the endoscopist has to briefly let go of the instrument shaft, which results in some loss of shaft control and "feel," with a tendency toward jerky insertion. Some endoscopists ingeniously compensate by fixing the colonoscope shaft between thigh and bed whenever the right hand is steering.

Occasional use of two-handed steering is entirely appropriate, but if the right hand is used too often for lateral angulations the endoscopist cannot torque-steer efficiently. Equally, if the right hand is away from the shaft for too long the endoscopist is being indecisive—it takes at most a second or two to make an angulation control adjustment and return the hand to shaft management.

"Single-handed" one-person colonoscopy

In "single-handed" colonoscopy, which we favor strongly, the endoscopist manages all aspects of the colonoscope control body (angulation controls, valves, and button switches) primarily with the left hand, leaving the right hand free to hold the shaft (Fig 7.21). This gives the endoscopist superior control and the opportunity to feel the colonoscope interacting with loops and bends.

• *Stance should be neutral, holding the colonoscope in a relaxed manner.* Colonoscopy mostly requires fine and fluent movements, like those of a violin player, so a similarly balanced position and handling are needed.

• *Grip the shaft (insertion tube) 20–30 cm away from the anus.* Many endoscopists make the mistake of holding too close to the anus, resulting in the need for frequent changes of hand-grip and jerky insertion technique. Holding the shaft further back makes for smoother insertion, easier application of torque (maintained twisting force), and better feel of the forces involved.

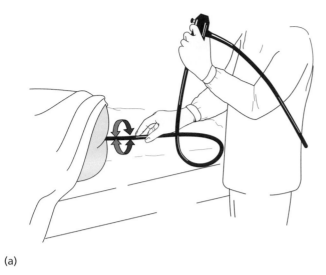

(a)

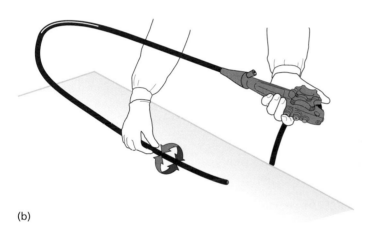

(b)

Fig 7.21 Single-handed maneuvering of the instrument shaft. The endoscope head is held in either (a) a comfortable position 60 degrees from vertical or (b) horizontally in the left hand, with the shaft supported on the bed in a "C position."

• *Hold the shaft in the fingers* to feel and manipulate the shaft deftly. A gauze or thin towel can be used for cleanliness and extra friction to avoid slippage from lubricant if required. A finger-grip (Fig 7.22, Video 7.7) is used for delicate movements and exact control (as for a key or a small screwdriver), as opposed to the clumsier fist-grip used for a hammer or large screwdriver. A finger-grip also makes it easier to feel whether the shaft is moving easily (is straight) or there is resistance (a bend or loop). Rolling the shaft between fingers and thumb allows shaft rotations of up to 360°, compared with a maximum of 180° achievable by wrist-twist.

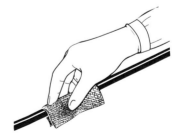

Fig 7.22 The instrument shaft is held delicately between the thumb and fingers (using a gauze for added friction if required).

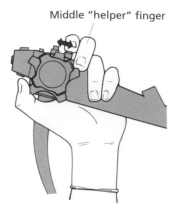

Middle "helper" finger

Fig 7.23 Single-handed control: the forefinger alone activates the air/water and suction valves; the middle finger is kept as "helper" to the thumb for major angulations.

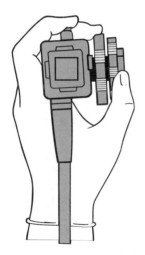

Fig 7.24 The thumb can reach the up/down and lateral angulation control if the left hand is positioned appropriately.

• ***Discipline the fingers of the left hand*** (Fig 7.23). Gripping the control body with only two fingers—the fourth (ring finger) and the little finger—lets the middle finger assume an invaluable role as "helper" to the thumb. Most endoscopists, unthinkingly but unnecessarily, use three fingers to hold the control body, and therefore find full angulation movements awkward. Single-handed steering is also made easier if the first finger alone operates the air/water or suction valves, which also leaves the middle finger free to help the thumb manage the angulation controls. The thumb can reach the up/down and lateral angulation control relatively easily, but some hand manipulation and change of grip is required for the middle finger to oppose the thumb on both controls. The grip that allows the thumb and middle finger to oppose needs to be practiced but, once mastered, allows complete control of the endoscope tip with one hand.

• The endoscope control head should be held in a relaxed position at around 60° to the vertical, although some endoscopists find holding the endoscope head horizontally more comfortable (Fig 7.21). Whatever approach is used, it is important to **keep the shaft of the instrument externally straight** so that torquing force is transmitted both down and up the shaft.

• ***Coordinate left- and right-hand activities.*** The endoscopist is like a puppeteer propelling a snake puppet by the tail, with control of its head and a view through its eyes, but scant idea of what is happening to the snake's body—because this is invisible within the abdomen. For single-handed endoscopy, in order to control the snake fluently and efficiently, each hand must be disciplined to fulfill its appropriate tasks. The left hand supports the control body, manages the air/water/suction valves and the up/down angulation control, and adds minor thumb adjustments of left/right angulation when needed (Fig 7.24). The right hand should provide the artistry of skilled colonoscopy, with sensory feedback as well as deft movements. Because the colon is a continuous series of short bends and convolutions, requiring multiple combinations of tip angulation and shaft movement and frequent air/water and suction valve activations, any small delays and uncoordinated movements rapidly summate, prolonging the procedure unnecessarily.

• ***Steer carefully and cautiously.*** Steering movements should be early, slow, and exact (rather than jerky and erratic). A slow start to each angulation movement allows it to be terminated within a few degrees if the result is tip movement in the wrong direction. A rapid steering movement in the wrong direction can lose the view altogether, and then tends to be ineffectually corrected by another large movement. Flailing around is unnecessary and inelegant. Each individual movement should be slow and intentional.

• ***Torque steering*** involves first angulating up or down as appropriate and then, rather than using the lateral angulation control knob, torquing (twisting, rotating) the instrument shaft clockwise or counterclockwise. This can be accomplished with the right hand. Alternatively, if the endoscope is held horizontally, with the shaft supported on the bed in a "C position," the larger muscles of the left arm can aid with torque steering when the endoscope shaft is straight (Fig 7.21b). Because the tip is angulated this rotation

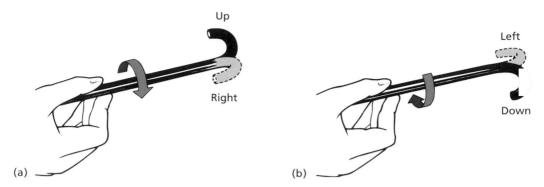

Fig 7.25 With a clockwise shaft twist: (a) an up-angulated tip moves toward the right, whereas (b) a down-angulated tip moves to the left.

should corkscrew it around laterally (Fig 7.25, Video 7.7), precisely, and quickly, and will often make use of the lateral angulation control unnecessary. Torque steering is, inevitably, affected by the direction in which the tip is angulated. "Up angulation" with clockwise torque moves the tip to the right, whereas it moves to the left if angulation is down. Torquing is also a valuable way of orienting the scope tip in order to suction fluid efficiently or target lesions accurately (Fig 7.19), thereby making biopsy-taking or polypectomy quicker and easier.

• *Torque steering only works when the shaft is straight* (Fig 7.26a). When a loop is present in the shaft, twisting forces applied to it will be lost within the loop (Fig 7.26b). With the shaft straight, twist becomes an excellent way to torque or corkscrew around bends. Twist is particularly useful if a bend is acute or fixed, when trying to push around will be likely to result in shaft looping rather than tip progress.

• *Torque control of a loop prevents torque steering.* The principles of loop control are discussed later in this chapter, when application of shaft torque force helps to straighten a spiral loop. Releasing "loop torque" (clockwise or counterclockwise) in order to "torque steer" in the other direction will allow the loop to re-form, but this can be avoided by making the required steering movement using the angulation controls.

• *Forceful angulation is ineffective.* With one angulation control fully angulated, applying the other control wheel only swivels the bending section very little, and scarcely affects the degree of angulation (Fig 7.27). On problem bends, therefore, concentrate on torque steering, because overforceful use of the lateral angulation control is likely to stress the angulation wires without improving the view or helping insertion.

Sigmoid colon—accurate steering

The sigmoid colon is an elastic tube (Fig 7.28a). When inflated it becomes long and tortuous; when deflated it is significantly shorter. When stretched by a colonoscope, especially if overinflated as well, the bowel inevitably forms both loops and acute bends (Fig 7.28b). However, it can also be shortened back, deflated, and telescoped

Fig 7.26 (a) Twist only affects the tip if the shaft is straight, (b) but it only affects the loop if one is present.

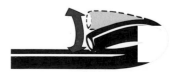

Fig 7.27 Lateral control angulation has little effect if the tip is maximally up- or down-angulated.

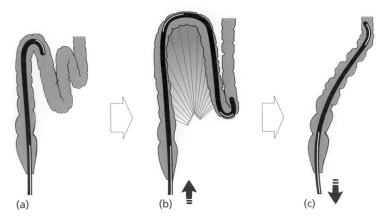

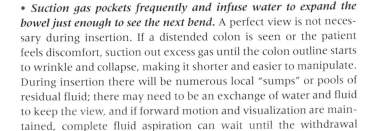

Fig 7.28 (a) The sigmoid colon is an elastic tube; (b) pushing causes loops but (c) pulling back shortens and straightens it.

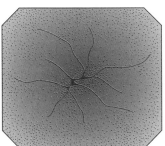

Fig 7.29 Aim at the convergence of folds.

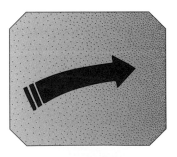

Fig 7.30 Aim at the darkest area.

into a few convoluted centimeters over the colonoscope (Fig 7.28c), just as a rolled-up shirt sleeve crumples over the arm.

• *Suction gas pockets frequently and infuse water to expand the bowel just enough to see the next bend.* A perfect view is not necessary during insertion. If a distended colon is seen or the patient feels discomfort, suction out excess gas until the colon outline starts to wrinkle and collapse, making it shorter and easier to manipulate. During insertion there will be numerous local "sumps" or pools of residual fluid; there may need to be an exchange of water and fluid to keep the view, and if forward motion and visualization are maintained, complete fluid aspiration can wait until the withdrawal phase. In the left lateral position fluid will quickly reaccumulate in the dependent sigmoid colon.

• *Insufflate gas or infuse water as little as possible.* A distended colon is less manageable and more uncomfortable than a nondistended one. The policy for gas or water distension, therefore, is "as much as necessary, as little as possible"; it is essential to see the colon but counterproductive to overdistend it. *Often the entire sigmoid colon can be intubated with water infusion alone, without the need for any gas insufflation.*

• *Bubbles should be avoided or removed.* They are caused by insufflating under water (angulate above it before insufflating, Fig 7.19) or by the detergent action of bile salts. Bubbles affect the accuracy of view but can be dispersed instantly by syringe-flushing 50 mL silicone emulsion anti-bubble solution down the instrument channel. Preparations used to avoid wind in babies are suitable for this purpose.

• *Use all visual clues.* A perfect view is not essential for progress but the endoscopist should be as sure as possible about the correct direction or axis of the colonic lumen, ascertained before pushing in. With only a partial or close-up view of the mucosal surface, there are usually sufficient clues to detect the luminal direction (Video 7.8):

– the lumen (when deflated, fluid-filled, or in spasm) is at the center of converging folds (Fig 7.29);

- aim toward the darkest (worst illuminated) area because it is furthest from the instrument and nearest the lumen (Fig 7.30);
- convex arcs are formed by haustral folds, or the wrinkling of circular muscles and the center of the arc indicates the correct direction in which to steer (Fig 7.31);
- in a capacious colon the muscle bulk of a tenia coli (Fig 7.32) can show as a longitudinal fold which, helpfully, follows the direction of the lumen.

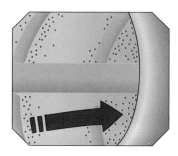

Fig 7.32 At acute bends a longitudinal bulge (tenia coli) shows the axis to follow.

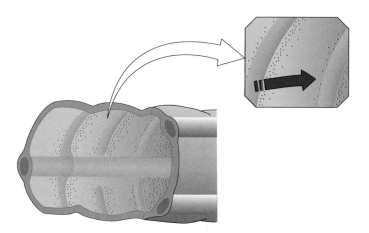

Fig 7.31 Aim at the center of the arc formed by folds.

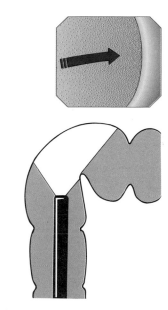

Fig 7.33 Endoscopic view of an acute bend, with a bright fold on the angle, and the "aerial" view.

- *Torque-steer, single-handed and cerebrally*. Each bend or haustral fold requires a conscious steering decision, but by combining up/down angulation and finger-grip rotation of the shaft, much of the sigmoid can be rapidly traversed with little or no use of the lateral angulation control. The angulated tip "corkscrews" efficiently, first one way and then the other, round the succession of bends or folds.
- *Concentrate on the monitor view* and suppress the normal social reflexes of looking at the patient or colleagues when talking to them. Acute bends or small polyps may disappear from view as the endoscopist looks away, and can take a surprisingly long time to find again.
- *Rehearse steering actions* before bends, while there is a "good" view. The give-away of a really acute bend may only be a bright angular fold seen against a darker background (Fig 7.33). Unlike the stomach, where there is usually sufficient room to see what is happening during steering maneuvers, colonic bends can be unforgivingly tight, so it is very easy to become unsighted and uncertain when angling around them. Before trying to pass an acute bend, suction any residual gas to partially collapse the bowel lumen (or utilize water infusion) and try out the best steering movements to use before becoming impacted. "Pre-steering" can allow the scope to enter an acute bend at a mechanical advantage (Fig 7.34).

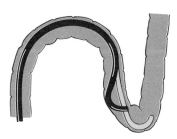

Fig 7.34 Pre-steer before pushing into an acute bend.

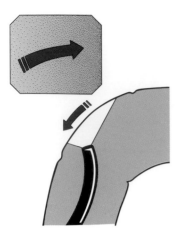

Fig 7.35 Pull back when lost—the mucosa slides away in the direction of the lumen.

• *If there is no view, pull back at once.* Pushing blindly, especially if there is a "red out" and total loss of view, is usually a pointless waste of time, and potentially a cause of perforation. If you are lost at any point in the examination, keep the angulation controls still or let them go entirely, then gently withdraw the instrument until the mucosa and its vessel pattern slips slowly past the lens in a proximal direction (Fig 7.35, Video 7.8). Steer toward the direction of slippage by angulating the controls or twisting the shaft, and the lumen of the colon should come back into view. Thrashing around blindly with the instrument rarely works; pulling back must help, for the bending section self-straightens if left free to do so. An expert "lost" for more than 5–10 seconds will admit it and pull back quickly to regain the view and re-orientate; the beginner flounders around in each difficult spot and is then surprised that the overall examination has taken so long.

• *Blind "slide-by" over the mucosa is occasionally permissible*, but only if unavoidable, for a few seconds and a few centimeters. The scope should slip easily over the surface, with the "slide-by" appearance of mucosal vascular pattern traversing the field of view. Only push on if this "slide-by" continues smoothly. If progress stops or causes the patient pain, stop at once, pull back, and try again. Force alone is rarely the answer during colonoscopy.

• *Try position change.* Changing the patient from the left lateral position to the back or right side not only lets gravity reposition fluid and gas, but also moves the colon, often with surprisingly beneficial results. A loop or bend that seems awkward or impassable with the patient in one position often becomes dramatically easier after position change (Fig 7.14, Video 7.6).

Endoscopic anatomy of the sigmoid and descending colon

The sigmoid colon is 50–70 cm or more in length when stretched by the instrument during insertion, although it will crumple down to only 30–35 cm when the instrument is straightened fully, which is why inspection is important during insertion, although it is desirable to keep the colon collapsed, shortened, and as straight as possible. The sigmoid colon mesentery is inserted in a V-shape across the pelvic brim, but is very variable in both insertion and length, and also quite frequently modified by adhesions from previous inflammatory disease or surgery. After hysterectomy the distal sigmoid colon can be angulated and fixed anteriorly into the space vacated by the uterus.

The colonoscope may stretch the bowel to the limits of its attachments or the confines of the abdominal cavity. The shape of the pelvis, with its curved sacral hollow and the forward-projecting sacral promontory, causes the colonoscope to pass anteriorly (Fig 7.36a) so that the shaft can often be felt looped onto the anterior abdominal wall before it passes posteriorly again to the descending colon in the left paravertebral gutter (Fig 7.36b). The result is that an anteroposterior loop occurs during passage of

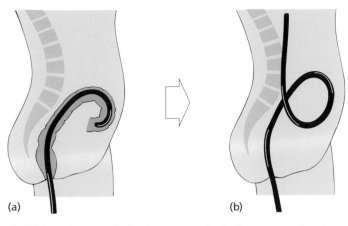

(a)   (b)

Fig 7.36 (a) The sigmoid colon loops anteriorly, (b) then passes up into the left paravertebral gutter.

the sigmoid colon and, since the descending colon is usually laterally placed, it tends to form a clockwise spiral loop (Fig 7.37, Video 7.9); the importance of this will be discussed later. When the sigmoid loop runs anteriorly against the abdominal wall it is possible to partially reduce or modify the sigmoid looping of the colonoscope (Fig 7.38). Pressure over the center of the abdomen directed toward the left lower abdomen with the hand (suprapubic area), when the straightened colonoscope tip is 20–30 cm from the anal verge, can help to reduce loop formation as the endoscope is advanced.

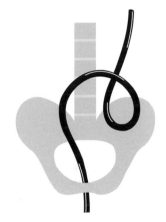

Fig 7.37 Sigmoid loop—anterior view (clockwise spiral).

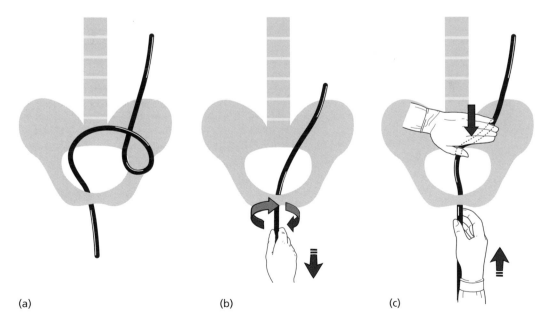

(a)   (b)   (c)

Fig 7.38 (a) A sigmoid spiral loop can be reduced with (b) clockwise torque and withdrawal followed by (c) hand-pressure over the central abdomen directed toward the left lower quadrant to restrict reformation of the loop on reinsertion.

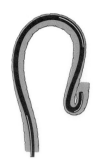

Fig 7.39 Fixed (iatrogenic) hairpin bend at the sigmoid-descending colon junction.

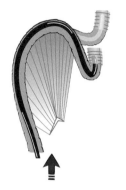

Fig 7.40 The length of the mesentery and the extent of retroperitoneal fixation determine the acuteness of the sigmoid–descending junction.

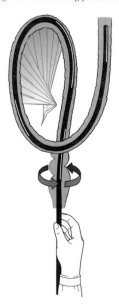

Fig 7.41 An alpha (clockwise) loop—a beneficial iatrogenic volvulus.

The descending colon is normally bound down retroperitoneally, so ideally runs in a fixed straight line, which is easy to pass with the colonoscope, except that there is often an iatrogenic acute bend at the junction with the sigmoid colon (Fig 7.39). This junction is only a theoretical landmark to the radiologist but, if the sigmoid colon is deformed upward by the colonoscope shaft, the resulting angulation becomes a very real challenge to the endoscopist. The acuteness of the sigmoid-descending angle depends on anatomical factors, including how far down in the pelvis the descending colon is fixed, but also on colonoscopic insertion technique. A really acute hairpin bend can result when the sigmoid colon is long or elastic enough to make a large "N loop" but retroperitoneal fixation of the descending colon happens also to be low in the pelvis (Fig 7.40). More often, when the sigmoid colon is long, an "alpha" spiral loop occurs, blessedly for both endoscopist and patient, because this avoids any acute angulation at the sigmoid-descending junction. The "alpha" describes the shape of the spiral loop of sigmoid colon twisted around on its mesentery or sigmoid mesocolon into a partial iatrogenic volvulus (Fig 7.41). Formation of the loop depends on the anatomical fact that the short inverted "V" base of the sigmoid mesocolon twists easily, providing that the sigmoid is long enough, there are no adhesions, and the descending colon is conventionally fixed.

Mesenteric fixation variations occur because of partial or complete failure of retroperitoneal fixation of the descending colon in utero. The result is persistence of varying degrees of descending mesocolon, which in turn has a considerable effect on what shape the colonoscope can force the colon into during insertion. The descending colon can, for instance, run up the midline (Fig 7.42) or allow a "reverse alpha" loop to form (Fig 7.43). Surgeons are well aware that there is great patient-to-patient variation in how easily the colon can be mobilized and delivered outside the abdominal cavity; occasionally the whole colon can be lifted out without

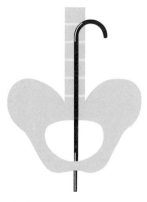

Fig 7.42 The endoscope may push a fully mobile distal colon up the midline to the diaphragm.

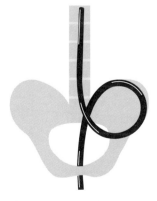

Fig 7.43 A reverse (counter-clockwise) alpha loop due to a persistent descending mesocolon.

dissection. A colon that is "easy" for the surgeon to mobilize is, however, often extremely unpredictable and "difficult" for endoscope insertion, because it is so mobile and can be pushed into atypical loops.

Sigmoid colon—the bends

Colons also vary greatly in elasticity and pain sensitivity—the sigmoid colon particularly. A degree of looping that is well tolerated by one patient may be unacceptably traumatic for another. The most challenging part of colonoscopy is to traverse the sigmoid as safely, gently, and rapidly as feasible. How best to achieve this depends on the anatomy and physiology of the individual patient, finessed by the equipment chosen and the endoscopist's hand skills and judgment.

Shorten acute or mobile bends by pulling back. Having angled around an acute bend, if the view is poor, gently pull back the hooked scope, which should simultaneously reduce the angle, shorten the bowel distally, straighten it out proximally, and disimpact the tip to give a better view (Fig 7.44). Because the colon can rotate on its attachments bends may change during such maneuvering, with any rotation being visible in close-up as a rotation of the visible vessel pattern (Fig 7.45). Watch the vessel pattern rotation carefully in close-up to know which direction to follow if a mobile bend rotates when pushing or pulling it.

The colonoscope will pass an acute bend more easily if:
• *the bend axis is oriented upward or downward* (easiest for thumb angulation)
• *the shaft is straight* (for more effective push)
• *the bowel is deflated slightly*
• *the bending section is not over-angulated* (to help it slide around).

Over-angulation, using both controls, tends to wedge the scope into a bend, making it unlikely to slide around. In the quest to get a better view around a difficult bend it is easy to forget this unproductive "walking-stick handle" effect (Fig 7.46).

Seeing the lumen doesn't always mean that it's safe to push. The acute angulation possible with modern endoscopes (Fig 7.28b) can mislead the endoscopist, giving a spuriously good view ahead when the bending section is jack-knifed and hopelessly impacted into an acute bend (such as the sigmoid-descending junction).

If in doubt . . . pull back.

Sigmoid colon—the loops

Colons vary hugely in length and attachments, with further constraints from surrounding organs and the limits of the abdominal cavity or any adhesions. Young men mostly have a short colon, unless constipated or with hemorrhoids. Women tend to have a longer colon, especially those with constipation. Longer colons allow more looping, but are often relatively pain insensitive (partly because the colon moves so easily), so the patient may suffer less than the endoscopist.

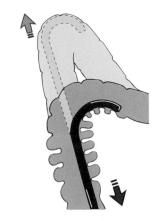

Fig 7.44 Pulling back flattens out an acute bend and improves the view.

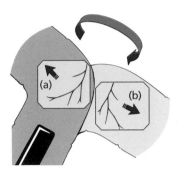

Fig 7.45 Rotation of the vessel pattern (from (a) to (b)) indicates rotation of the colon, so the endoscopist needs to change steering direction too.

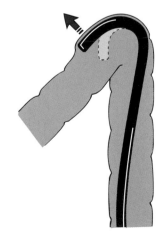

Fig 7.46 De-angulate at the splenic flexure to avoid "walking-stick handle" impaction.

Sigmoid looping of some degree is unavoidable as the scope pushes up the apex of the sigmoid colon (Video 7.10).

Clues suggesting that a loop has formed are:

• *loss of the "one-to-one" relationship* between the amount of shaft being inserted through the anus and the movement inward of the scope tip;

• *squeezing discomfort*, which is the commonest warning of looping and is acceptable only when the discomfort is mild and the scope tip is advancing with minimal resistance;

• *"paradoxical movement,"* in which the instrument tip slides outward as the shaft is pushed in (or vice versa), which suggests a substantial loop;

• *resistance* to insertion of the scope shaft is encountered, which is best felt with the finger-grip;

• *the angulation controls feel "jammed up."* As the scope loops, increasing friction in the wires from the angulation controls to the bending section causes the controls to feel stiffer and stiffer, but with less and less steering effect;

• *the length of scope inserted is greater than expected* for the anatomical location.

Inexperienced endoscopists often do not notice these clues, can become deaf to patient protest (or overgenerous with sedation), and think that forceful management of the colonoscope is "normal." Colonoscopy should (mostly) be a deft and gentle procedure, manageable by finger-grip and fine movements.

Instrument stretch pressure into a loop feels like "wind" or the "urge to go." The patient should be warned before using force and whenever pushing begins to cause looping or discomfort (e.g. "you will feel some wind pain for a few seconds, but there is no danger"). Uncomfortable pushing should be limited to a tolerable time— ideally no more than 20–30 seconds. Looping pain stops at once when the instrument is withdrawn slightly, so there is no excuse for long, continued periods of pain, even in examinations where recurrent loops form.

Abdominal hand-pressure can be helpful, but only when the sigmoid happens to loop anteriorly, close to the abdominal wall (Fig 7.38), which is especially likely in a protuberant abdomen. The assistant compressing nonspecifically over the lower abdomen, which opposes the sigmoid loop, may reduce stretch pain and can make the scope slide around more easily. Assistant hand-pressure is only relevant during the 20–30 seconds needed to resist looping during inward scope-push. There is no need to fatigue the assistant by asking for more prolonged hand pressure, especially as the sigmoid loop is nowhere near the abdominal surface in around 50% of patients.

Gently "pushing through" the sigmoid colon is allowable, providing it is easy and requires no undue force. Using careful steering combined with "persuasive pressure" the scope may slide around the bends of the sigmoid and up into the descending colon (Fig 7.47).

Inward pushing should be applied gradually, avoiding sudden thrusts. Shorter sigmoid loops require more subtlety and often

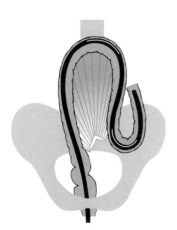

Fig 7.47 A very long sigmoid may allow the scope to "push though" and avoid forming a hairpin bend.

cause more pain, as their short mesenteric attachments are restrictive and stretch force is more localized and obvious. Pushing is most likely to be effective in a longer colon, which tends to accommodate to the instrument, letting it slide in more freely with no acute bends and more likelihood of favorable (spiral) loops.

It is dangerous to ignore pain and to push into a loop when the scope tip is jammed and not progressing.

Short or pain-sensitive colons—pull back and straighten to avoid an "N"-loop

Although some degree of looping is inevitable as the instrument pushes inward, in a short colon the endoscopist may, by subtlety, water infusion, repeatedly pulling back, avoiding insufflation, and deflating whenever possible, be able to achieve virtually "direct" passage from sigmoid to descending colon with minimal stretch (Fig 7.48). This is elegant technically and comfortable for the patient.

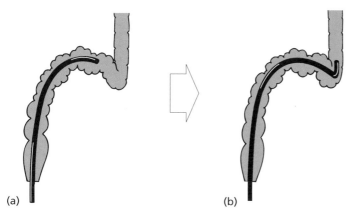

(a)   (b)

Fig 7.48 (a) Pull back and deflate to keep the sigmoid short, (b) which may allow direct passage to the descending colon.

Upward "N"-looping of a short colon is the classic loop of colonoscopy, as originally seen on fluoroscopy and thought of as a flat loop resembling the letter N. Whatever its actual configuration, "N"-looping tends to cause the scope tip to approach the sigmoid-descending junction at an acute angle or hairpin bend (Fig 7.49), but this can potentially be straightened back so that the instrument is able to slide directly (and painlessly) up the descending colon (Video 7.11).

At the sigmoid-descending junction the scope enters retroperitoneal fixation, so it is a good place to try to pull back and get control of the sigmoid loop while the tip and bending section are fixed. Direct passage straight up the descending colon is the ideal, trying to steer the tip around the junction without forcing up the sigmoid loop. This takes subtlety, and even experts can have trouble in achieving it, pulling back gradually, torquing (usually clockwise), and steering cautiously (usually with a poor view). Typically, a less skilled endoscopist, having slid around the sigmoid with panache,

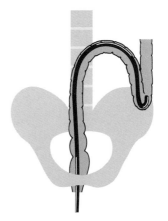

Fig 7.49 An "N"-loop stretching up the sigmoid colon.

will have stretched up a large (iatrogenic) sigmoid loop (Fig 7.50a) and so created an acute hairpin bend and extra difficulty as a result. Being more careful, using water to minimally distend, using less push, and then withdrawing gradually with clockwise (usually) torque (Fig 7.50b), using tip steering to maintain luminal view, can be rewarded by "direct" passage from the sigmoid to descending colon (Fig 7.50c). Repositioning the patient from the left lateral position to their back or right side can help to open a tight sigmoid-descending (and rectosigmoid) junction (Fig 7.14). Dynamic position change can be used proactively to help optimize configuration of the colonic anatomy to help open tight corners or help control loops.

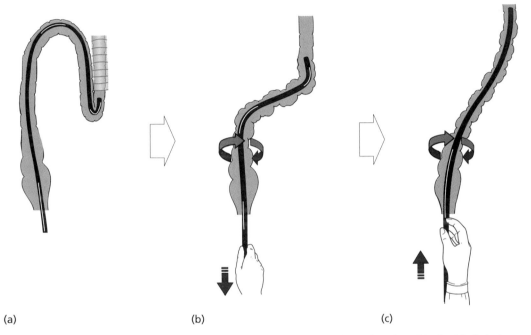

(a)   (b)   (c)

Fig 7.50 (a) An "N" loop with the tip hooked into the retroperitoneal descending colon: (b) pull back with clockwise torque to reduce the loop, maintaining a luminal view; (c) when the scope feels maximally straightened (sometimes "blind"), redirect the tip and push in maintaining clockwise torque.

There can be a useful "N-spiral" element because most sigmoid loops run in a clockwise spiral—anteriorly out of the pelvis, over the pelvic brim, then curving laterally and posteriorly into the descending colon (Fig 7.36). The resulting spiral shape can be used by a single-handed endoscopist to corkscrew directly around (with strong clockwise torque) into the descending colon, with a minimum of push force, and so no relooping (Fig 7.51, Video 7.11).

A pain-sensitive colon suggests trying this "short-scope" "N-spiral" approach. Pulling back and deflating during insertion around the sigmoid and taking extra care (and time) to withdraw, torquing clockwise and trying to straighten at the sigmoid-descending junction (see the following steps) will often achieve direct painless passage into the descending colon. This largely explains why the technique of some endoscopists allows them to perform successful colonoscopy with little or no sedation while others routinely rely on heavy sedation or anesthesia.

At the sigmoid-descending junction try the following steps:

1 *Pull back the shaft* to reduce the loop, which creates a more favorable angle of approach to the junction and also optimizes the instrument mechanics (Fig 7.48).

2 *Deflate* (without losing the view) to shorten the colon and make it as pliable as possible.

3 *Change the patient to supine or right lateral position* (Fig 7.14). This can improve the view of the sigmoid-descending junction (air rises, water falls) and may sometimes also cause the distal descending colon to drop down into a more favorable configuration for passage.

4 *Pull back with clockwise torque* in the hope that corkscrewing force will direct the angulated tip into the descending colon and hold it there (Fig 7.51). Successful "pull-with-clockwise-twist" uses this tip fixation, together with scope withdrawal, to shorten ("pleat," "accordion," "concertina") the sigmoid over the colonoscope shaft, while simultaneously sliding the tip up the descending colon. Sometimes the act of pulling causes the hooked tip to impact into the mucosa (Fig 7.50b). Careful angulation control is needed, any wrong move being likely to lose the critical retroperitoneal tip fixation and cause the instrument to fall back into the sigmoid. When the maneuver is successful (Fig 7.50c) the endoscopist has the warm feeling of "getting something for nothing," passing directly into descending colon without looping or pain.

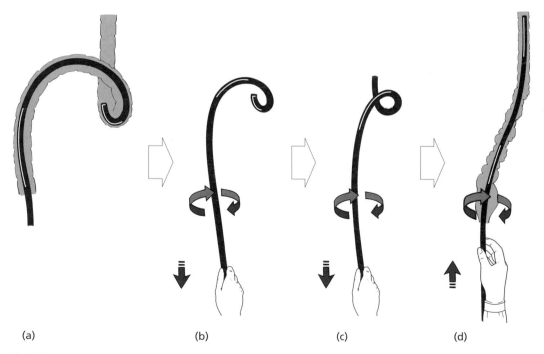

(a)   (b)   (c)   (d)

Fig 7.51 (a) An "N"-spiral loop with the tip at the sigmoid-descending junction: (b) torque clockwise and withdraw gradually; (c) keep torquing and find the lumen of the descending colon; (d) then push in (still torquing forcibly to prevent relooping).

5 *Water exchange and/or immersion* can be helpful to weigh down and de-angulate the colon to facilitate passage.

6 *Consider abdominal pressure.* The assistant pushes over the central abdomen toward the left lower abdomen so as to compress the loop or reduce the abdominal space. Sometimes additional counterpressure is applied with the left hand in the left iliac fossa to move the sigmoid-descending junction medially.

7 *"Pushing through" the loop should be the last option and only if the scope moves forward with acceptable levels of force.* If the scope tip remains static despite push, the sigmoid may be severely angulated or fixed; stopping the colonoscopy should be considered, as alternative colonic imaging would be safer and avoid the risk of adverse events. If pushing through the loop, the patient should be warned that some brief discomfort may occur. It may sometimes be better to warn the patient and push in calculatedly rather than struggling with repeated failed attempts at shortening. A few seconds (typically 10–15) of careful "persuasive pressure" may slide the instrument tip around the bend and then allow straightening again.

Suspect a long N-spiral or alpha loop if insertion seems easy. If, during insertion, no particularly acute flexure is encountered in the sigmoid colon and the instrument appears to be sliding in a long way without problems or acute angulations, it is possible that a long N-spiral or alpha loop is being formed (Video 7.12). If so (especially if confirmed on fluoroscopy or the magnetic imager), push on to the proximal descending colon or splenic flexure before trying any withdrawal/straightening maneuver. Even if the patient has mild stretch pain, reassure them and continue, steering carefully until the tip has passed through the fluid-filled descending colon to the splenic flexure, reached at about 90 cm (rather than 50 cm as expected with a straight scope) (Fig 7.52). Straightening back halfway round a long N-spiral or alpha loop is a mistake, as this may cause the spiral/alpha configuration to rotate back into a shorter N-loop configuration, which then results in greater difficulty in reaching the descending colon (alternatively, it may fall back, require reinsertion, and so prolong the uncomfortable insertion phase).

A long sigmoid colon tends to push into a spiral loop. A spiral loop can occur in around 60% of patients; in 10% the spiral is flat against the posterior abdominal wall in "alpha" shape, as originally described with the patient lying flat for X-ray fluoroscopy (Fig 7.53). Using the magnetic or 3D imager allows loops to be assessed from the lateral as well as anteroposterior view (Fig 7.54a,b and Video 7.13), showing a much greater frequency of spiral configuration. Any spiral loop is a blessing, since the shape means that there is no acute bend between the sigmoid and descending colon so that, with continued gentle inward pushing (Fig 7.54c) the scope can slide relatively easily into the descending colon with no resistance, before being straightened (Fig 7.54d).

It may take several attempts to create a spiral loop. Inserting around a long and tortuous sigmoid the endoscopist may struggle to disimpact the scope tip from several acute angulations, but the act of doing so can reposition the colon into spiral shape, with sudden

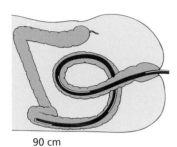

90 cm

Fig 7.52 In an alpha loop the scope runs through the fluid-filled descending colon to the splenic flexure at about 90 cm (posterior view—as for the endoscopist).

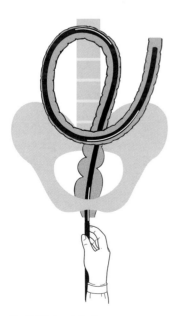

Fig 7.53 An alpha loop.

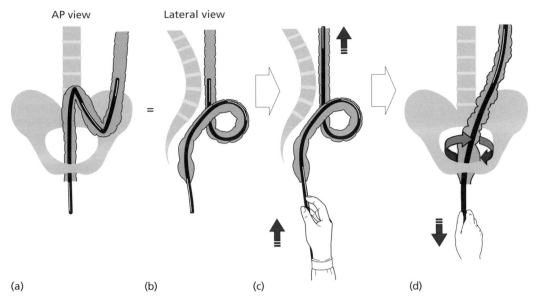

Fig 7.54 Many "N"-loops (a), if also seen in lateral view (b), are actually "N-spiral" loops, so (c) advance toward the splenic flexure before (d) gradually withdrawing with clockwise torque to straighten the colon.

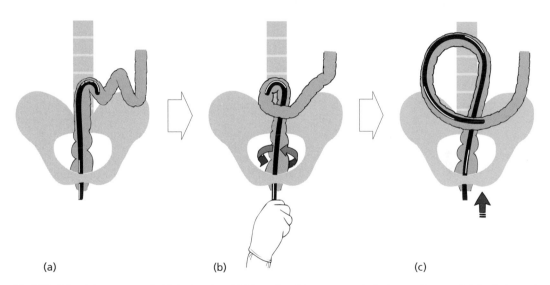

Fig 7.55 "The alpha maneuver": (a) during sigmoidal insertion, (b) try counterclockwise rotation to point the tip toward the cecum and (c) push in to form an alpha or spiral loop.

improvement of view and the opportunity for successful progress. This process of (gently) bullying the colon to produce a spiral loop was historically called "the alpha maneuver" (Fig 7.55). It typically involved counterclockwise twisting force under X-ray control and helped insertion of early colonoscopes, which had limited angulation characteristics so as to protect their fragile glass-fiber bundles. The concept of encouraging spiral loop configuration, or of making

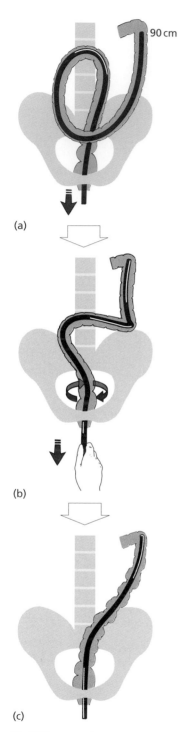

(a)

(b)

(c)

Fig 7.56 (a) An alpha loop (b) derotates with clockwise torque and withdrawal (c) to straighten completely.

the most of the opportunity when it occurs spontaneously, remains a valuable option even with modern instrumentation (especially if the magnetic imager is available for guidance).

Straightening a spiral loop

A spiral or alpha loop must be removed at some stage, usually before pushing around the splenic flexure, to avoid stressing the patient and scope. Most colonoscopists prefer to straighten out the loop (to 50 cm) as soon as the upper descending colon or splenic flexure is safely reached (at 90 cm) and then to pass around the flexure with a straightened instrument. However, every colonoscopist has also experienced the chagrin of seeing the tip slide back when a straightening attempt is made too early, before the tip is adequately fixed by friction or angulation. It can occasionally be better in an unusually long but mobile colon to pass around the splenic flexure into the transverse colon with the spiral loop still in place before attempting reduction.

Spiral loop straightening is simply an exaggerated version of the "pull back and twist" maneuver described previously, combining withdrawal with strong clockwise torque to remove the loop in a few seconds (Fig 7.56, Videos 7.9–7.14). Withdrawing the shaft initially reduces the size of the loop and makes derotational twisting easier. Torque alone would change the sigmoid spiral into an "N" shape but not straighten the loop. By combining the two actions simultaneously, pulling back and torquing the whole instrument, the loop is smoothly and easily removed to 50–60 cm—often in only 2–3 seconds and with obvious improvement of the "feel" as the shaft straightens. The clockwise torque used should push the tip inward toward the splenic flexure. Any tendency to slip back is prevented by applying more twist and less pull, or by hooking the tip more actively into the splenic flexure. Such twisting forces do not harm the colonoscope.

Derotation should be easy and atraumatic. If straightening the loop proves difficult or the patient has discomfort, the situation should be reassessed. Do not use excessive force. The sigmoid loop that has formed may not be a clockwise spiral loop but a "reversed alpha" (see "Atypical sigmoid loops and the 'reversed alpha'" below). In the absence of a magnetic imager, the endoscopist must judge this by feel (and results).

Longer colons—the S-loop

When "pushing through" a very long sigmoid colon, a flat S-shaped loop may form with no spiral configuration (Video 7.14), so twist has no effect when pulling back to straighten it. The key to success is to push on to the splenic flexure, angulating around it to fix the tip before removing the loop.

Atypical sigmoid loops and the "reversed alpha"

"Atypical" spiral loops can form when colon attachments are unusually mobile, particularly those of the descending colon (see "Distal colon mobility and 'reversed' looping" below). The colonoscope may force a mobile colon into a counterclockwise spiral, or

even a complex mix of clockwise and counterclockwise loops. In practical terms this variation should make little difference to the endoscopist, except for the need to apply the correct derotational force when pulling back to straighten. A counterclockwise "reversed alpha" loop (Fig 7.43) may allow the scope tip to slide up into the descending colon as easily as a conventional spiral loop, with no obvious clue that there is anything odd or unusual. As around 90% of sigmoid loops spiral clockwise, the unsuspecting endoscopist can waste time and make things worse by trying to derotate the atypical (counterclockwise) loop with conventional clockwise torque. If a magnetic imager is being used, the configuration and its solution are obvious. If relying on shaft feel and guesswork, try counterclockwise torque if the sigmoid appears not to be straightening. Occasionally derotational torque has to be first one way, then the other.

Remove shaft loops external to the patient

Straightening colonic loops may result in shaft loops external to the patient. The mechanical construction of an endoscope, with its protective wire claddings and four angulation wires, means that any shaft loop increases the resistance of the instrument to twisting/torquing movements. Looping also decreases tip angulation by causing friction in the angulation wires. For this reason, shaft loops are mechanically undesirable even when they occur outside the patient. The shaft should run in an easy curve to the anus, without unnecessary bends. Any loops forming outside the patient should ideally be derotated and straightened. This is easily done by rotating the control body to transfer the loop to the umbilical (which can accommodate up to three loops without harm to its internal structures) (Fig 7.57 and Video 7.15). Sometimes it may be necessary to unplug the light guide connector from the light source and then unravel the umbilical. The alternative for the dexterous endoscopist is to derotate the external shaft loop by twist, while steering the tip into the lumen, the straightened colonoscope rotating on its axis.

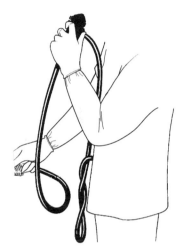

Fig 7.57 Shaft loops forming outside the patient can be transferred to the umbilical by rotating the control head.

Diverticular disease

In severe diverticular disease there may be a narrowed lumen, pericolic adhesions, and problems in choosing the correct direction (Fig 7.58a). However, once the instrument has been laboriously inched through the area, the "splinting" effect of the abnormally rigid sigmoid may facilitate the rest of the examination by preventing any sigmoid loop from re-forming. The secret in diverticular disease is extreme patience, with care in visualization and steering combined with greater than usual use of withdrawal, rotational, or corkscrewing movements. It helps to realize that a close-up view of a diverticulum means that the tip is at right angles to the lumen and must be deflected or withdrawn to find the lumen, which is often deformed and unobvious (Fig 7.58b).

Using a thinner and more flexible pediatric colonoscope or gastroscope may make an apparently impassable narrow, fixed, or

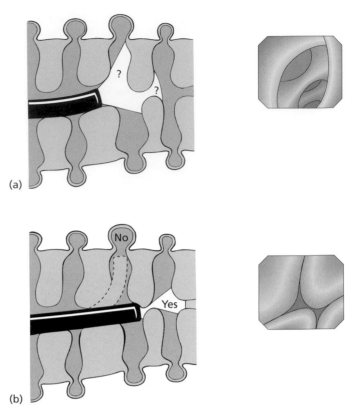

Fig 7.58 (a) Choosing the correct path can be difficult in diverticular disease:
(b) a circular view is a diverticulum—the lumen will be at 90°, and often
squashed.

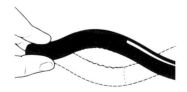

Fig 7.59 If the tip is fixed it cannot
be steered (the shaft moves instead).

angulated sigmoid colon relatively easy to examine, which sometimes also saves the patient from surgery.

Having successfully passed severe fixed or angulated sigmoid
diverticular disease (especially if it has taken a short scope to do so),
it becomes the endoscopist's worst nightmare if the proximal colon
then proves to be long and mobile.

If the tip is fixed or impacted, it cannot be steered. The tip and
bending section of a flexible endoscope normally angulates because
it is free to move easily. If the tip is fixed, attempted angulation
simply moves the shaft around instead (Fig 7.59). This is an inher-
ent limiting factor of flexible endoscopes, and is why the endoscopist
may be unable to steer effectively in fixed diverticular disease or to
get a proper view in a tight stricture. Torque is less affected in such
situations, which is another reason torque steering is so useful.

Use of water infusion is particularly helpful in patients with very
hypertrophic musculature and redundant mucosal folds. Water can
distend a narrow segment better than air, having the combined
advantages of being noncompressible, remaining in the dependent
sigmoid colon (rather than air's tendency to rise and distend only
the proximal colon), and holding the mucosal folds away from the
lens for an improved close-up view. The water may also help reduce
frictional resistance when passing an angulated or fixed colon.

Be prepared to abandon the procedure if postoperative or diverticular adhesions have fixed the colon, making passage impossible or dangerous. If there is difficulty, if the instrument tip feels fixed and cannot be moved by angling or twisting, and the patient complains of pain during attempts at insertion, there is a danger of perforation, and the attempt should be abandoned. Sometimes a different endoscope (e.g. pediatric colonoscope or gastroscope) or another endoscopist may succeed. Only a very experienced colonoscopist with very good clinical reasons should put the patient and instrument at risk under these circumstances; usually the most experienced are the most prepared to stop and refer for CT colonography.

Descending colon

The descending colon can be a 20 cm long "straight" and traversed in a few seconds. For the gravitational reasons described above, when the patient is in the left lateral position there is characteristically a horizontal fluid level (Fig 7.60, Video 7.16). Often there is sufficient air interface above the descending colon fluid (or blood in emergency cases) to allow the scope to be steered above it. If opaque fluid makes steering difficult, it may be quicker, rather than wasting time suctioning, to turn the patient onto their back or right side to fill the descending colon with air (Fig 7.14). Apart from this positional trick, and the frequent use of clockwise torque or occasionally hand pressure to minimize sigmoid colon re-looping, no particular skills or maneuvers are needed in the average descending colon. In a long colon the descending may be so tortuous that the endoscopist, having struggled through a number of bends and fluid-filled sumps, believes the scope has arrived in the proximal colon when it has only reached the splenic flexure.

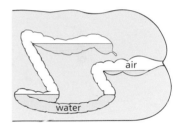

Fig 7.60 Fluid levels in the left lateral position.

Distal colon mobility and "reversed" looping

If the descending colon is mobile, without retroperitoneal fixation, the normal anatomy can disappear. At the most extreme, the colonoscope may run through the "sigmoid" and "descending" distal colon straight up the midline (Fig 7.42), inevitably resulting in a "reversed splenic flexure" and consequent mechanical problems later in the examination. The endoscopist is alerted to this when counterclockwise rotation seems to help insertion at the sigmoid-descending junction. This indicates that an unconventional counterclockwise spiral loop or "reversed alpha" has been formed by the instrument (Fig 7.43), with the corollary that other oddities may occur during insertion. The endoscopist can use counterclockwise torque to push the mobile descending colon outward against the lateral margin of the abdominal cavity. This regains the conventional configuration so that the instrument runs medially (rather than in reverse) around the splenic flexure, and is able to adopt the favorable "question-mark" shape to reach the cecum. Such apparently mysterious manipulations become understandable under fluoroscopic control or with the magnetic imager.

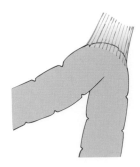

Fig 7.61 The phrenicocolic ligament.

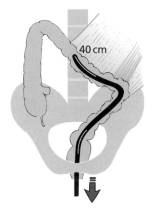

Fig 7.62 The splenic flexure can pull back to 40 cm if there is a free phrenicocolic ligament.

Splenic flexure

Endoscopic anatomy

The splenic flexure is where the colon angulates medially and anteriorly beneath the left costal margin, inaccessible to hand pressure. The position of the flexure is variably fixed according to the degree of mobility of the fold of peritoneum—the phrenicocolic ligament—which attaches it to the diaphragmatic surface (Fig 7.61). In some subjects the splenic flexure is tethered high up into the left hypochondrium, but in others it is relatively free and can be pulled down toward the pelvis (Fig 7.62). A lax phrenicocolic ligament, a common feature of long, mobile colons, makes control of the transverse colon more difficult by depriving the endoscopist of any fixed point or fulcrum with which to exert leverage during withdrawal maneuvers (the cantilever effect). The configuration of the splenic flexure is also affected by the patient's position, principally because of the effects on it of the transverse colon, which sags down under gravity in the left lateral position, making the flexure acute (Fig 7.63a), or pulls it open in the right lateral position (Fig 7.63b).

Insertion around the splenic flexure

The splenic flexure is the "half-time" point of colonoscopy, where the instrument should straighten back to 50 cm from the anus. This ensures that the colonoscope is under proper control before tackling the proximal colon. The commonest reason for experiencing problems in the proximal colon is because the colonoscope has been inadequately straightened at the splenic flexure. Persistence of loops makes the rest of the procedure progressively more difficult or impossible. If the splenic flexure is passed with straight shaft configuration (at 50 cm), using the above rules, the rest of colonoscopy insertion should usually be finished within a minute or two.

Anyone who frequently finds the proximal colon or hepatic flexure difficult to traverse should apply the "50 cm rule" at the splenic flexure, and is likely to find most of the problem solved, because the distal colon has been properly straightened.

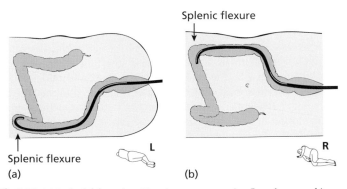

Fig 7.63 (a) In the left lateral position the transverse colon flops down, making the splenic flexure acute, (b) whereas in the right lateral position (or supine) gravity rounds off the flexure and makes it easier to pass.

Passage around the apex of the splenic flexure is usually obvious when the instrument emerges from fluid into the air-filled, often triangular, transverse colon (Fig 7.64, Video 7.17). However, while the flexible and angulated bending section of the colonoscope passes around without effort, the stiffer segment at around 10–15 cm in the leading part of the shaft may not follow so easily. This problem is accentuated in the left lateral position, because drooping of the transverse colon causes the splenic flexure to be acutely angled (Fig 7.63a) compared with its configuration when opened out by gravity in the supine or right lateral position (Fig 7.63b). Difficulty getting around the splenic flexure is often due to sigmoid buckling (Fig 7.65) or to formation of a "walking-stick handle" or "hockey stick" deformity (raising the splenic flexure on its mesentery toward the diaphragm).

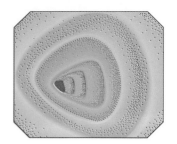

Fig 7.64 The transverse colon is usually triangular.

To pass the splenic flexure without force or re-looping:

1 Straighten the scope. Pull back with the tip hooked around the flexure until the instrument is around 50 cm from the anus (the distance can be 40–60 cm according to mobility of the flexure or angulation around it). This straightens any sigmoid loop, pulls down the flexure, and rounds it off *(NB splenic avulsions or capsular tears have been reported, so be gentle)*.

2 De-angulate the tip. Full "bending-section" angulation results in such acute angling that it tends to impact in the splenic flexure, preventing further insertion (the "walking-stick handle" or "hockey stick" effect). Having obtained a view of the transverse colon and pulled back, consciously de-angulate the tip a little so that the instrument runs around the outside of the bend (Fig 7.46), even if this means worsening the view somewhat.

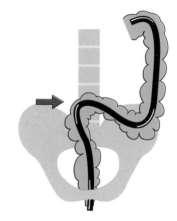

Fig 7.65 Sigmoid colon buckling.

3 Deflate the colon (suction) slightly to shorten the flexure and make it malleable.

4 Use clockwise torque on the shaft. As explained above, the clockwise spiral course of the sigmoid colon from the pelvis to its point of fixation in the descending colon means that applying clockwise torque to the colonoscope shaft tends to counteract any looping tendency in the sigmoid colon while pushing in (Fig 7.66). Clockwise torque will only be effective to keep the shaft straight if any significant looping has first been removed by pulling back, and if the descending colon is normally fixed. Because the tip is angulated, applying clockwise shaft torque may affect the luminal view into the transverse colon, and readjustment of the angulation controls may be needed to redirect the tip.

5 Counterclockwise torque may be needed as you cross the splenic flexure. As the splenic flexure tends to rotate anteriorly, using counterclockwise torque helps elevate the distal transverse colon and de-angulate the flexure.

6 Change patient position and try again. As pointed out earlier, the left lateral position used by most endoscopists has the undesirable effect of causing the transverse colon to flop down (Fig 7.63a) and make the splenic flexure acutely angled. Turning the patient onto their back or right side has the opposite effect. The transverse colon sags to the right side and, together with gravity, often pulls the splenic flexure into a smooth curve without any apparent "flexure" at all (Fig 7.63b).

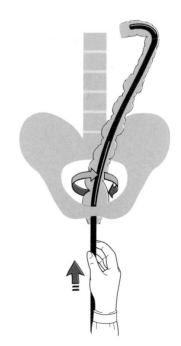

Fig 7.66 Torque clockwise while advancing to keep the sigmoid straight.

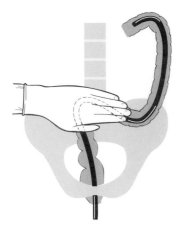

Fig 7.67 Control sigmoid looping by hand-pressure to help pass the splenic flexure.

7 *Apply assistant hand-pressure* over the sigmoid colon to help prevent re-looping (Fig 7.67). Any resistance encountered at the splenic flexure is likely to result in stretching upward of the sigmoid colon into an "N"-loop or spiral loop, which dissipates more and more of the inward force applied to the shaft if the loop increases. It is immediately obvious to the single-handed endoscopist that such a loop is forming, because the "one-to-one" relationship between insertion and tip progress is lost; in other words, the shaft is being pushed in but the tip moves little or not at all. Pull back again to restraighten the shaft if this occurs.

8 *Asking the patient to breathe in and hold their breath* for a few seconds as the endoscope is advanced can be helpful, as this lowers the diaphragm and can help to de-angulate the flexure.

9 *Push in, but slowly.* The instrument tip cannot advance around the splenic flexure without some degree of inward push. So, as well as clockwise torque, continued gentle inward pressure is needed (aggressive pushing simply re-forms the sigmoid loop). All that is needed for success is firm inward pressure on the shaft, which causes very gradual inward slippage of the tip into the transverse colon. While pushing, deflate again, and make any necessary compensatory steering movements. A combination of these various maneuvers may help the tip slide around the splenic flexure, using the angulation controls to "squirm" the bending section and the suction valve to collapse the bowel.

10 *If a variable stiffness scope is being used, stiffen it.* Once the splenic flexure is reached and the instrument is straightened, stiffen the shaft (the effect starts 30 cm from the tip, the leading part remaining flexible) to stop the sigmoid region from buckling (Fig 7.67) or re-looping and facilitate inward pushing to slide the tip around the flexure. Once the leading part of the shaft is safely into the transverse colon, however, *unstiffen* the instrument again to allow the rest of the shaft to slide around the flexure more easily.

11 *Water immersion* may also be useful to help de-angulate the flexure.

12 *If it does not work, try a different position, pull back and start again.* If the tip is not progressing from the amount of shaft being inserted it is obvious that a sigmoid loop is re-forming, pull back and run through all the above actions again before pushing in once more. It may take two or three attempts to achieve success.

Strategies to help navigate the splenic flexure include:
1. Pull back to straighten the scope (to around 50 cm)
2. De-angulate the tip
3. Deflate the colon (suction)
4. Use clockwise, or occasionally counterclockwise, torque on the shaft to prevent sigmoid looping
5. If the shaft is straight and the scope tip around the splenic flexure is pointing toward the left side (anteriorly), consider counterclockwise torque to reorient the direction of the tip to the right (posteriorly)
6. Change patient position to the back or right side
7. Apply assistant hand-pressure
8. Ask the patient to breathe in and hold for a few seconds
9. Push in, but slowly
10. Stiffen a variable scope
11. Consider water immersion
12. If it does not work, try a different position, pull back, and start again

The "reversed" splenic flexure

Atypical passage around the splenic flexure is seen to occur in about 5% of patients if imaging is available. The instrument tip passes laterally rather than medially around the splenic flexure, because the descending colon has moved centrally on a mesocolon (Fig 7.68, Video 7.17). This is of more than academic interest because, having passed laterally round the flexure and displaced the descending colon medially, the advancing instrument forces the transverse colon down into a deep loop. The instrument is then mechanically under stress and difficult to steer, and the hepatic flexure is approached from below at a disadvantageous angle, making it difficult to reach the cecum and virtually impossible to steer into the ileo-cecal valve. With a reversed splenic loop, even when the instrument tip can be hooked onto the hepatic flexure, the sheer bulkiness of the reversed loop configuration actively holds down the transverse loop, stopping it being straightened and lifted up into the ideal "question-mark" shape.

De-rotation of a reversed splenic flexure loop may be possible and will avoid these problems later in the examination. This can be done by torquing strongly counterclockwise (rather than the usual clockwise torque), usually after withdrawing the tip toward the splenic flexure. The subsequent examination is so much quicker, and also more comfortable for the patient, that the time spent doing this can be well worthwhile. Counterclockwise de-rotation makes the tip pivot around the phrenicocolic suspensory ligament and swing medially (Fig 7.69a). After that, by maintaining counterclockwise torque while pushing in, the instrument can be made to pass across the transverse colon in the usual configuration, forcing the descending colon back laterally against the abdominal wall (Fig 7.69b).

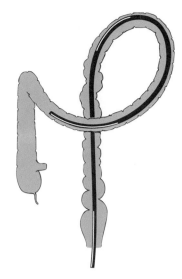

Fig 7.68 A "reversed" splenic flexure will result in a deep transverse loop.

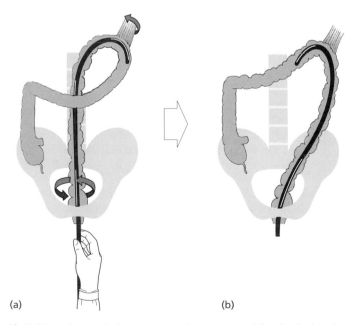

(a)   (b)

Fig 7.69 (a) Counterclockwise rotation (b) swings a mobile colon back to the normal position.

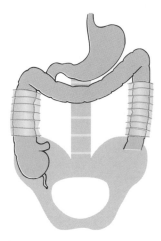

Fig 7.70 The transverse colon is anterior, over the duodenum and pancreas. The descending and ascending colon are fixed retroperitoneally.

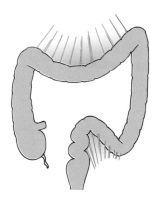

Fig 7.71 Colon mesenteries—the transverse and sigmoid mesocolons.

Counterclockwise straightening is most easily performed under imaging (Video 7.17) but is also quite feasible by feel, using these guidelines and a little imagination whenever atypical looping is suspected in the proximal colon. A reversed splenic flexure/mobile descending colon is one reason for an unexpectedly difficult colonoscopy. Sometimes the best solution, if the problem is suspected but imaging is not available and attempts at counterclockwise de-rotation have failed, is simply to get a move on and to "push through," accepting the fact that tip control will be suboptimal in the right colon. For the reasons given above, if a reversed splenic loop is present, it is rare to be able to enter the ileum without successful de-rotation and straightening, because the looped and stressed instrument will not angulate sufficiently. If ileoscopy is essential and a reversed loop is present it is likely to be necessary to pull the instrument out to 50 cm at the splenic flexure, attempt counterclockwise de-rotation, and pass in again. Failing to do this and simply trying to angulate the tip forcibly into the ileum is likely to stress the bending section and not succeed.

Transverse colon

Endoscopic anatomy

In 30% of subjects the transverse colon lies anteriorly just beneath the abdominal wall, held forward by the vertebral bodies, the duodenum, and pancreas, and relates to the left and right lobes of the liver (Fig 7.70). It is enveloped in a double fold of peritoneum called the transverse mesocolon (Fig 7.71), which originates from the posterior wall of the abdomen and hangs down posterior to the stomach, varying considerably in length. In a barium enema study, the transverse colon of 62% of erect females drooped down into the pelvis, compared with only 26% of males. This longer transverse "U" loop largely accounts for the 10–20 cm greater mean colon length found in women despite their smaller stature (total colon length was 80–180 cm) and probably also contributes to our experience that 70% of difficult colonoscopies are in women (previous hysterectomy making only a small contribution). The depth to which the transverse colon can be looped downward by

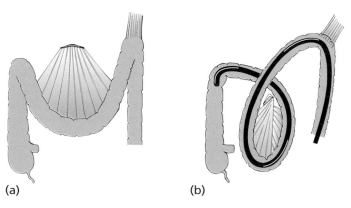

(a)   (b)

Fig 7.72 (a) Transverse mesocolon. (b) A gamma loop.

colonoscope pressure also affects the angle at which the endoscope approaches the hepatic flexure, in the same way that the size of the sigmoid colon loop causes an acute sigmoid-descending colon bend. Because the transverse mesocolon (Fig 7.72a) is broad-based it is relatively unusual for a *"gamma" loop* to form (Fig 7.72b).

The triangular configuration of the transverse colon (Fig 7.64 and Video 7.18) depends on the relative thinness of the circular muscles compared with the three longitudinal muscle bundles or teniae coli (Fig 7.73). In some patients (such as those with long-standing colitis, but also some normals) the circular musculature is thicker and the transverse colon can be tubular. Both at the mid-transverse flexure and at the hepatic flexure a true "face-on" view of the haustral folds may be obtained. These present a characteristic "knife-edge" or "ladder" appearance (Fig 7.74); it is therefore easy to confuse the mid-transverse flexure with the hepatic flexure. The mid-transverse bend should be less voluminous, show no blue/gray liver patch, and may show transmitted cardiac (double) or aortic (single) pulsation. It can also be distinguished by imaging, local palpation of the anterior abdominal wall, or transillumination (if the room is darkened).

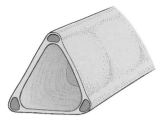

Fig 7.73 The triangular configuration is due to the three teniae coli.

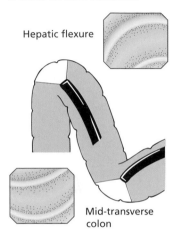

Fig 7.74 Similar "knife like" haustra are seen at the mid-transverse colon and hepatic flexure.

Insertion through the transverse colon

Insertion around the transverse should be easy, **unless** the sigmoid colon has also looped, thus reducing inward force transmission. In the mid-transverse colon, however, the angled scope tip often forms a surprisingly sharp bend, pushing a transverse "U" loop downward into the pelvis. A drooping transverse colon, frequently found in women and those with a long colon, inevitably results in greater friction resistance to passage; the force required then results in secondary sigmoid looping as well. This combination can be a major problem for "push and go" endoscopists who have not learned the wisdom of shortening and controlling colon loops (Video 7.19). Measures to counteract forming a transverse "U" loop include suctioning to deflate and shorten the colon, supine positioning, deep inspiration, or abdominal pressure with a transverse lift.

The longitudinal fold of the ante-mesenteric tenia coli may bulge into a voluminous transverse colon, which is a useful pointer to the correct axis—rather like the white line down the center of a road (Fig 7.75). Appreciating this is particularly helpful at very acute angulations, as occurs when the mid-transverse colon is pushed down by the endoscope; a tenia coli can be followed blindly to push or angulate round the bend and see the lumen beyond (Fig 7.76).

After passing the mid-point of the transverse, it may be slow and difficult, with considerable push-pressure needed, to "climb the hill" up the proximal limb of the looped transverse colon (Fig 7.77a, Video 7.20). In most patients this aggressive approach can be avoided if the transverse colon can be shortened by deflating it and pulling back. The tip, being hooked around the mid-transverse angulation of the "U" loop, then lifts up and flattens the transverse (Fig 7.77b) so that the tip advances as the shaft is withdrawn. This is the phenomenon of "paradoxical movement." Hand-pressure upward from the lower abdomen to lift up the transverse loop can often be very helpful to help advance the tip of the instrument by

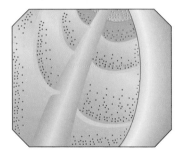

Fig 7.75 The longitudinal bulge of a tenia coli shows the axis of the colon.

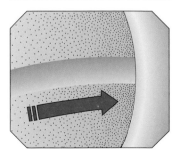

Fig 7.76 Follow the longitudinal bulge (tenia coli) round an acute bend.

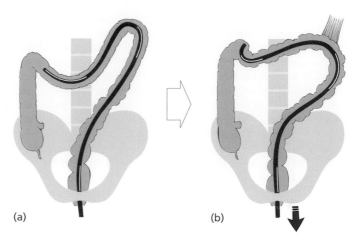

(a)

(b)

Fig 7.77 (a) If the passage up the proximal transverse colon is difficult, (b) hook around the angulation of the transverse "U" loop and pull back to lift and shorten it.

reducing the loop. If there are problems, change of position (usually to supine, sometimes to right lateral, left lateral, or even prone) can also help (Fig 7.14).

When the tip is established in the proximal transverse colon, *counterclockwise torque* often helps it to advance toward the hepatic flexure. This useful phenomenon results from a flattening out of the counterclockwise spiral formed by the shaft running anteriorly and medially around the splenic flexure from the descending colon to the transverse colon (Video 7.20).

In the transverse colon—to reach the hepatic flexure:
1. Pull back to lift up the transverse loop
2. Deflate
3. Try counterclockwise torque
4. Try upward abdominal hand-pressure to "lift" the transverse
5. . . . and supine positioning

A mobile splenic flexure may adversely affect "transverse lift" maneuvers. The fulcrum or cantilever effect caused by the phrenicocolic ligament which fixes the normal splenic flexure is crucial. In some patients this attachment is lax, allowing the splenic flexure to be pulled back to 40 cm (rather than the usual 50 cm rule) (Fig 7.78a); the colon is then found to be hypermobile and unresponsive to any of the normally effective withdrawal or twisting movements (Fig 7.78b). When this occurs the use of force is ineffectual, but deflation, counterclockwise torque, upward hand-pressure to "lift" the transverse, posturing (usually in left lateral but sometimes to right lateral), and gentle perseverance will coax the tip up to the hepatic flexure. Simple aggression and force usually worsen the loop, whereas subtlety and patience often win.

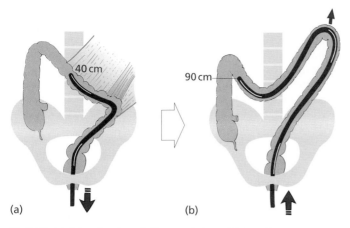

Fig 7.78 (a) If the phrenicocolic ligament is lax, withdrawal maneuvers are ineffective, (b) and pushing in simply re-forms the "U" loop.

A gamma loop may form in a very long redundant transverse colon (Fig 7.79), as can be well seen using the magnetic imager (Video 7.21). A gamma loop is large and rarely removable, both because of its sheer size (conflicting with the small intestine and other organs during attempted de-rotation) and because colon mobility makes it difficult to find any point where angulation will anchor the tip. The instrument therefore falls back each time it is withdrawn and it is necessary to push on to the cecum with the loop in place. This can make cecal/ileal intubation challenging.

On the rare occasions that a gamma loop is successfully removed, this is by combined withdrawal and very strong torque (usually counterclockwise) to lift up the transverse colon into a more conventional position. Prone positioning can sometimes help to prevent the loop from recurring. Having the magnetic imager available greatly increases the chance of success, because it shows very obviously which direction of torque to apply, and whether the de-rotation maneuver is starting to work. Using the magnetic imager, it is also sometimes possible to prevent a gamma loop, torquing strongly counterclockwise while crossing the splenic flexure and early transverse colon. Another option for removing a gamma loop is to attempt loop removal once the tip is secured within the terminal ileum. Here the tip is anchored and provides sufficient purchase to de-rotate the loop with strong counterclockwise torque.

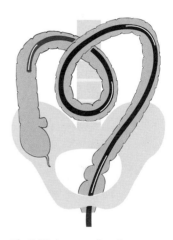

Fig 7.79 A gamma loop in a redundant transverse colon.

Hand pressure over the transverse or sigmoid colon

Hand pressure is helpful in well over 30% of transverse colons, reducing the tendency for scope looping within the abdominal cavity and encouraging as straight a line as possible to the hepatic flexure and cecum. The rationale for pressure in the lower left abdomen over the looping sigmoid colon has been described (Fig 7.67), and the tendency of the sigmoid to re-loop at all stages of the examination has also been mentioned. Because of this

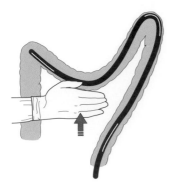

Fig 7.80 "Specific" hand pressure can be used to elevate the transverse colon for deep transverse "U" loops.

tendency, hand pressure over the sigmoid colon is a good bet whenever the instrument is looping (even in the transverse), and its application has therefore been called *"nonspecific" hand pressure*.

Brief and gentle upward hand pressure to "lift" the transverse can be quite helpful, provided that it passes close enough to the abdominal wall to be accessible. This maneuver has been called *"specific" hand pressure*. This can be applied to help advance the tip of the instrument by reducing the transverse "U" loop, or, more ideally, once the loop has been reduced to help prevent re-looping as the endoscope is advanced across the transverse colon. In the proximal colon, at any time that a few extra centimeters of insertion are needed but cannot be achieved, try abdominal hand pressure—first try "specific" pressure, according to the results of local palpation, but, if all else fails, use "nonspecific" pressure (in the left lower abdomen).

> *In the transverse colon, try "specific" hand pressure upward in either the:*
> * Mid abdomen (to counteract and "lift" the sagging transverse colon; Fig 7.80)
> * Left hypochondrium region (to push the whole loop toward the hepatic flexure)
> * Right hypochondrium (to impact directly on the hepatic flexure)

Hepatic flexure

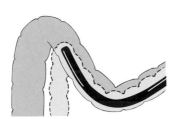

Fig 7.81 Aspirate to shrink the hepatic flexure toward the scope.

The hepatic flexure (Video 7.22) is, from both an anatomical and endoscopic viewpoint, a nearly 180° hairpin bend, similar in many respects to the bend at the sigmoid-descending junction but more constant in its fixation and more voluminous.

Passing the hepatic flexure

1 *Assess from a distance* the correct direction around the flexure because, after the tip reaches into it, it is so close to the opposing mucosa that it is very difficult to steer except by a predetermined plan. At all costs avoid impacting the tip forcibly against the opposing wall or it will catch in the haustral folds and there will be no view at all.

2 *Aspirate air carefully* from the hepatic flexure, to collapse it toward, but not actually onto, the tip as it moves around (Fig 7.81).

3 *Ask the patient to breathe in* (and hold their breath), which lowers the diaphragm, and often the flexure too.

4 *Steer the tip blindly in the previously determined direction* around the flexure. As the hepatic flexure is very acute, it takes some confidence to angulate nearly 180° around in the same direction without seeing well (Fig 7.82). Use both angulation controls simultaneously to achieve full angulation; adding clockwise torque may be helpful.

5 *Counterclockwise torque* with scope advancement may also help by reducing the transverse colon loop.

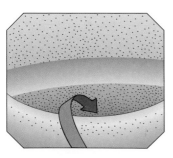

Fig 7.82 Suction toward, then angle acutely (180°) around the acute hepatic flexure.

6 *Left lateral positioning* may be helpful to open up the flexure.

Passing the hepatic flexure:
1. Watch carefully
2. Deflate
3. Patient breathes in
4. Steer blindly around in predetermined direction
5. Use counterclockwise torque
6. Left lateral patient positioning is helpful

---

7 *Withdraw the instrument* substantially with torque (usually clockwise), using tip steering to maintain luminal view, for up to 30–50 cm to "lift" the transverse colon and straighten out the colonoscope (Fig 7.83a,b) for passage into the ascending colon.

8 *Try upward abdominal hand-pressure* to "lift" the transverse colon.

9 *Aspirate air again* once the ascending colon is seen, in order to shorten the colon and drop the colonoscope down toward the cecum (Fig 7.83c).

Dropping down into the ascending:
1. Pull back scope with clockwise torque
2. Consider hand pressure to "lift" the transverse
3. Deflate
4. Bingo!

A combination of these maneuvers is used simultaneously. Aspiration brings the hepatic flexure toward the tip until the inner fold of the flexure can be passed, the colonoscope is withdrawn (either by manipulation of the shaft or by the endoscopist pulling the colonoscope outward, using both hands simultaneously to

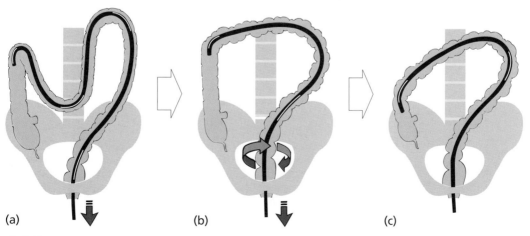

(a)   (b)   (c)

Fig 7.83 (a) When around the hepatic flexure and viewing the ascending colon, (b) pull back with clockwise torque to straighten, maintaining a luminal view, (c) and aspirate to collapse the colon and pass toward the cecum.

work the angulation controls), and the tip is steered maximally around until it can be sucked down into the ascending colon. A parallel has already been drawn between the "hook, withdraw, and clockwise twist" situation in the transverse loop and hepatic flexure and the "right twist and withdrawal" method of shortening the sigmoid N-loop at the sigmoid-descending colon angle. The same instrument maneuvers apply to both, except that they must be exaggerated at the hepatic flexure because of its larger dimensions.

Position change

Position change is another trick that helps coax the colonoscope tip into and around the hepatic flexure. The left lateral position is the best for passing the hepatic flexure; however, one can try changing the patient's position (to a supine, prone, or sometimes even right lateral position) if there is difficulty in passing in left lateral position (Fig 7.14). Using brute force at the hepatic flexure rarely pays off, since the combined sigmoid and transverse colon loops can take up most of the length of even a long colonoscope shaft. With the instrument really straightened at the hepatic flexure, only about 70 cm of the shaft should remain in the patient (this is one of the situations where a distance check helps to ensure that the colonoscope is straight and results in easy and painless insertion).

Is it the hepatic flexure—or might it be the splenic?

A final, embarrassing, point is that if things are not working out at the hepatic flexure after applying the various tips, the colonoscope may actually still be at the splenic flexure. In a redundant colon it is possible to be overoptimistic and get hopelessly lost. The clue to this is often that the hepatic flexure (in left lateral position) is dry or air-filled, whereas the splenic is likely to be fluid-filled.

Ascending colon and ileo-cecal region

Endoscopic anatomy

The ascending colon is posteriorly placed at its origin from the hepatic flexure, but then runs anteriorly so that where it joins the cecum it is just under the anterior abdominal wall and usually accessible to finger palpation or transillumination. In 90% of subjects, the ascending colon and cecum are predictably fixed retroperitoneally, but the remainder may be mobile on a persistent mesocolon, with correspondingly variable positions.

The cecum is an evolutionarily defunct and stagnant part of the colon proximally, between the point of entry of the ileo-cecal valve and the appendix orifice. It is typically about 5 cm in length, but sometimes surprisingly capacious and difficult to examine properly. Being out of the normal stream, the cecum is often poorly prepared and may require irrigation for proper views. The *cecal sling fold*, well known to surgeons, typically results in anterior angulation of the cecum. This angulation is why the cecum and appendix may be poorly seen from the ascending colon and why position change (to partially prone, supine, or right lateral) can help the scope slide toward the cecal pole and appendix.

At the pole of the cecum the three teniae coli may fuse around the appendix (crow's-foot or "Mercedes Benz sign"; Fig 7.84), but the anatomy is somewhat variable. Between the teniae coli and the marked cecal haustra there can be cavernous outpouchings, which are difficult to examine.

The appendix orifice is normally an unimpressive slit, which is often crescentic because the appendix is folded around the cecum. As the appendix is characteristically flexed toward the center of the abdomen, it can give guidance as to the likely site of entry of the ileum (see "Finding the ileo-cecal valve" below). Only rarely is the appendix orifice seen straight-on as a tube, probably when the cecum is fully mobile. The appendix may sometimes be less than obvious at the center of a local whirl of mucosal folds—not unlike a Danish pastry. The operated appendix usually looks no different unless it has been eradicated entirely or invaginated into a stump, when it can sometimes resemble a polyp (take care—perhaps take a biopsy but do not attempt polypectomy!).

The ileo-cecal valve (Video 7.23) is on the prominent ileo-cecal fold encircling the cecum about 5 cm back from its pole. Unfortunately for the endoscopist, the orifice of the valve is often a slit on the invisible upstream or "cecal" aspect of the ileo-cecal fold. The most the endoscopist normally sees is the slight bulge of the upper lip. It is therefore rare to see the orifice directly without specific close-up maneuvers.

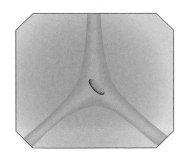

Fig 7.84 Appendix orifice at the fusion of the three teniae coli.

Reaching the cecum

On seeing the ascending colon the temptation is to push in, but this usually results in the transverse "U" loop re-forming and the tip sliding back. The secret is to deflate. The resulting collapse of the capacious hepatic flexure and ascending colon will drop the tip downward toward the cecum (Fig 7.83c); it also lowers the position of the hepatic flexure relative to the splenic flexure and, with this mechanical advantage, pushing inward should become more effective. Aspirate and steer carefully down the center of the deflating lumen, then push the last few centimeters into the cecum. If it proves difficult to reach the last few centimeters to the cecal pole, change the patient's position to semi-prone (even a partial position change of 20–30° may help) or, if that does not work, change to a supine or right lateral position (or even prone). Once in the cecum, the bowel can be reinflated to get a better view. The right lateral position generally helps to open up the cecum and drain fluid from the area, improving the view.

The cecum can be voluminous with pronounced haustral infoldings and a tendency to spasm, making it confusing to examine. In particular, it is possible to be mistaken about whether the pole has actually been reached. One catch is that the ileo-cecal valve fold, the major circumferential fold at the junction of the ascending

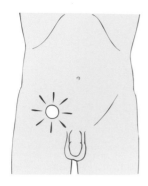

Fig 7.85 Transillumination deep in the iliac fossa suggests the cecum.

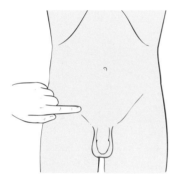

Fig 7.86 Finger-pressure in the right iliac fossa indents the cecum.

colon and the cecum—on which is situated the give-away bulge of the valve—has a tendency to be in tonic spasm. The contracted fold may easily be mistaken by the unwary either for the appendix orifice or for the ileo-cecal valve. Insufflating and pushing in with the instrument tip and/or using *extra IV antispasmodic* medication will reveal the cavernous cecal pole beyond.

Be careful to identify landmarks before assuming "total colonoscopy" has been performed. The appendix orifice and ileo-cecal valve should be identified as positive landmarks and photodocumented. "Soft" but suggestive evidence is given by seeing right iliac fossa transillumination (Fig 7.85) or finger-palpation indenting the cecal region (Fig 7.86). At the same time the colonoscope should, after withdrawal, be at 70–80 cm. The cecal pole is often difficult to examine, not always completely clean, and sometimes in tonic spasm; a "too good to be true" appearance may, therefore, actually be only the ascending colon (or even the hepatic flexure). Inability to locate the ileo-cecal valve opening and noting that the shaft distance on withdrawal is only at 60–70 cm should warn of this possibility.

Finding the ileo-cecal valve
The "appendix trick" or "bow and arrow" sign (Video 7.23), as described by JD Waye, is an ingenious way of finding the ileo-cecal valve and simultaneously entering the ileum too—a "double whammy" when it works the first time.
1 *Find the appendix orifice* (Fig 7.87a).
2 *Imagine an arrow* pointing in the direction of the appendix lumen (Fig 7.87b).
3 *Angulate in that direction and pull back* slowly (still angled) for about 3–4 cm (Fig 7.87c).
4 At this point *expect the proximal lip of the ileo-cecal valve to start to ride up over the lens*, with shiny bumps of close-up ileal villi apparent, rather than the mirror-smooth crypt-spotted colon mucosa.

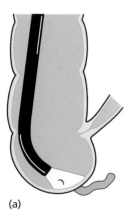

(a)

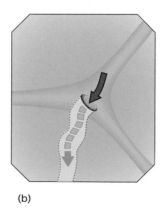

(b)

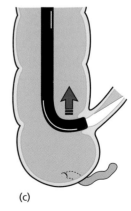

(c)

Fig 7.87 (a) Angle in the direction of the appendix lumen (b), and (c) pull back until the proximal lip of the ileo-cecal valve rides up into the view.

5 *Slowly insufflate and twist or angulate gently to wangle into the* *ileum.* Change of patient position to the supine or right lateral (or even prone) may be helpful if the initial view of the valve is poor or disadvantageous for tip entry.

Entering the I-C valve ("the appendix trick"):
1. Find appendix
2. Imagine bow and arrow
3. Angulate in that direction
4. Pull back slowly
5. Insufflate
6. Consider patient position change to supine or right lateral

---

The "appendix trick" succeeds when (as is usual) the appendix is bent toward the center of the abdomen, from which direction the ileum also enters the cecum. The appendix effectively acts as an indicator of direction (rather as an airport windsock indicates wind direction).

The other way to find the valve is to pull back about 8–10 cm *from the cecal pole* and to look for the first prominent circular haustral fold, around 5 cm back from the pole. On this "ileo-cecal" fold will be the telltale thickening or bulge of the ileo-cecal valve. A common mistake is to look for the valve when the endoscope tip is in the cecal pole, rather than pulling back to the mid-ascending colon to get a proper overall view from a distance. Looking at this ileo-cecal fold, with the cecum moderately inflated, one part of it should be seen to be less perfectly concave than the rest. It may be simply flattened out, bulge in (especially on deflation when it often bulges more obviously and may bubble or issue ileal contents), show a characteristic "buttock-like" double bulge, or, less commonly, have obvious protuberant lips or a "volcano" appearance (Fig 7.88). It is rather uncommon to see the actual slit orifice or pouting lips of the valve straight on, because the opening is normally closed.

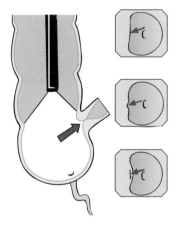

Fig 7.88 The ileo-cecal valve is a bulge on the ileo-cecal fold—a flattening, single, or double bulge or a "volcano."

Entering the ileum
"Direct entry" into the ileum is made easier by a combination of *actions.*

1 *Rehearse at a distance* (about 10 cm back from the cecal pole) the easiest steering movements, preferably combining shaft twist and down-angulation to point the tip toward the valve (Fig 7.89a). If possible, rotate the endoscope so that the valve lies in the downward (6 o'clock) position relative to the tip, because this allows entry with an easy downward angulation movement (lateral or oblique movements are more awkward single-handedly) and because the tip air outlet is situated below the lens, but needs to enter the valve first in order to open up the ileum with insufflation.

2 *Pass the colonoscope tip* in over the ileo-cecal valve fold in the region of the valvular bulge.

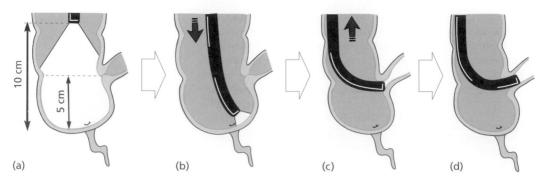

(a)   (b)   (c)   (d)

Fig 7.89 (a) Locate the ileo-cecal valve, (b) insert beyond, angulate, and deflate slightly, (c) pull back if required until the "red-out" is seen, (d) and insufflate to open the valve.

3 *Angulate the scope tip toward the valve* (Fig 7.89b). Overshoot a little, so that the action of angulation directs the tip into the opening, not short of it.

4 *Deflate the cecum partially* to make the valve supple (Fig 7.89b).

5 *Pull back the scope if required*, angling downward until the tip catches in the soft lips of the valve, resulting in a "red-out" of transilluminated tissue (Fig 7.89c), typically with the telltale granular appearance of the villous surface in close-up (as opposed to the pale shine of colonic mucosa).

6 *On seeing the "red-out," freeze all movement.*

7 Then *insufflate CO_2/air* to open the lips (Fig 7.89d) and wait, gently twisting or angling the scope a few millimeters if necessary, until the direction of the ileal lumen becomes apparent. If considerable angulation has been used to enter the valve, *de-angulation* may be needed to straighten things out and let the tip slide in.

8 *Multiple attempts may be needed for success*, both in locating the valve and entering the ileum, if necessary rotating to slightly different parts of the ileo-cecal fold, hooking over it and pulling back to pass the area repeatedly. On each successive attempt try to learn from the problems of the previous one, refining down tip movements to a centimeter or two and a few degrees either way.

9 *Change of patient position* to the supine or right lateral position (or even prone) may also help to open up the cecum and remove fluid to improve visualization of the valve.

10 *An underwater approach* can facilitate intubation. Completely aspirate all air from the cecum and infuse water until the valve is fully underwater. This relaxes the valve such that it opens to allow passage inward facilitated by more water infusion and gentle probing with the scope tip. This "underwater" approach is particularly effective if a cuff or distal attachment is on the scope.

11 *The biopsy forceps can be used as a guidewire.* If only a distant, partial, or uncertain view can be obtained of the ileal bulge or opening, it is possible to use the biopsy forceps to locate and then pass into the opening of the valve (Fig 7.90), either to obtain a blind biopsy or to act as an "anchor." The forceps fix the position of the tip relative to the valve and facilitate endoscope passage through it (as with a guidewire). Even if entry into the ileum is not intended,

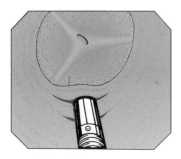

Fig 7.90 The biopsy forceps can be used to locate the slit of the valve, and then pass into it.

the opened forceps can be used to hook back the bulge of the upper lip of the valve to visualize the ileal opening and make identification certain.

Entering the I-C valve (direct approach):
1. Look for valve bulge
2. Push in over it
3. Angulate tip toward the valve
4. Deflate
5. Pull back, if required
6. Insufflate
7. Consider patient position change to supine or right lateral
8. Underwater approach may be helpful
9. Can use biopsy forceps as a guidewire

Entry into the ileum can be in retroflexion. This "last-ditch" maneuver is only likely to work in a capacious colon and if the scope is completely straightened and responsive. It is a useful option when the ileo-cecal valve is slit-like and invisible from above (Fig 7.91). Retrovert the tip to visualize and then enter the valve from below but only do this if the scope retroverts easily as there is a risk of perforation, particularly with a larger-diameter scope (Fig 7.92a). Very acute angulation of the colonoscope tip is needed, with maximum up/down and lateral angulation, and often some twist of the shaft as well. Fairly forceful inward push may be needed to impact low enough in the cecal pole to visualize the valve. The extra length of the bending section of video endoscopes, due to the CCD electronics, means that in a normal-sized colon the tip retroverts into mid-ascending with no view of the valve so this technique is easier and safer with a pediatric scope or one with a tight bending section rather than with a standard adult scope.

In those few cases that the valve can be seen, pull back to impact the tip within it (Fig 7.92b), insufflate to open the lips, and de-angulate and pull back further to enter the ileum, with or without use of the forceps (Fig 7.92c).

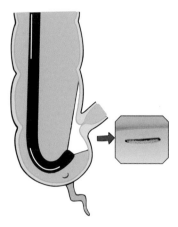

Fig 7.91 A slit-like valve may only be visible in retroversion (in a large colon).

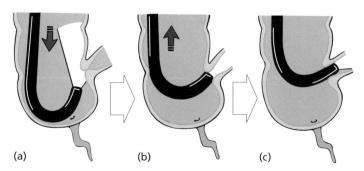

(a)   (b)   (c)

Fig 7.92 (a) If necessary, retroflex to see the valve, (b) pull back to impact, (c) and insufflate and de-angulate to enter the ileum.

Problems in entering the ileo-cecal valve occur for a number of reasons. The endoscope may be in the hepatic flexure, not the cecum. Even if the tip is in the right place, the chosen "bulge" on the ileo-cecal valve fold may not be correct; some valve openings are entirely flat and slit-like (Fig 7.93a), effectively invisible on the reverse side of the fold. It is a mistake to aim the objective lens (at the center of the endoscope tip) exactly at the slit, which may result in impaction of the scope tip against the upper lip of the valve (Fig 7.93b). This is why overshooting the opening slightly (Fig 7.93c) will let the angled tip edge into the ileum successfully, even though the initial view has been less good.

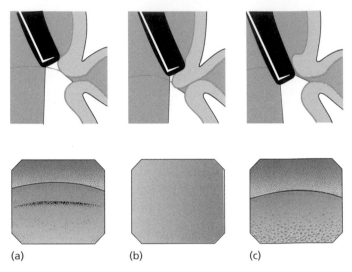

(a)   (b)   (c)

Fig 7.93 Entering the ileo-cecal valve. (a) Distant view of the valve slit. (b) Pushing in directly may impact against the upper lip. (c) Overshooting the valve lets the tip angulate in successfully.

Those cases of active inflammatory disease (especially Crohn's) where the colonoscopist wants to see the terminal ileum are also those where the valve is most likely to be narrowed and, although a limited view may be possible and biopsies taken, the valve may be impassable. Conversely, in some cases of longstanding, chronic, or healed previous colitis, the valve may be atrophic and widely patent, without the usual soft or bulging lips. Endoscopists who perform lower endoscopic procedures on pediatric patients should aim to complete an ileocolonoscopy unless the procedure is being performed for a specific indication that does not require this.

Inspecting the terminal ileum

The terminal ileum surface looks granular in air, but under water the villi float up prettily—like coral or lambs' wool. The ileal surface is often studded with raised lymphoid follicles resembling small polyps, or these can be aggregated into plaque-like Peyer's patches. Sometimes the ileum is surprisingly colon-like, with a pale shiny surface and visible submucosal vascular pattern. After colon resection the difference between colon and ileum may be imperceptible because of villus atrophy. Using dye spray (0.1% indigo carmine) or blue light imaging to highlight the surface detail will rapidly discriminate between the granular or "sandpaper" appearance of the ileal mucosa and the small circumferential grooves of the colonic surface, which give a "fingerprint" effect.

The ileum is soft, peristaltic, and collapsible compared with the colon. Rather than attempting forceful insertion, greater distances can be traversed by gentle steering and deflation, so that the intestine collapses over the colonoscope. At each acute bend it is best to deflate a little, hook round, pull back, and then steer gently (if necessary, almost blindly) around and inward before pulling back again to relocate the direction of view—a "two steps forward and one step back" approach that applies throughout colonoscopy. When the colonoscope tip is in the ileum, it can often be passed in up to 30–50 cm with care and patience, although this length of intestine may be folded on to only about 20 cm of instrument. Air distension in the small intestine should be kept to a minimum because it is particularly uncomfortable and slow to clear after examination—another reason for routinely using CO_2.

Overtubes and balloon colonoscopy

A stiffening overtube, sometimes called a "splinting device," is almost never used now, but may hold a looping sigmoid colon straight and allow easier passage into the proximal colon. The original extremely stiff (wire-reinforced) overtubes for colonoscopy had disadvantages that discouraged most endoscopists from using them. The tube had to be on the instrument before starting (or the endoscope completely withdrawn before putting it on), and insertion was sometimes traumatic, with perforations reported.

"Balloon colonoscopy" is the modern equivalent technique. The double-balloon approach incorporates two balloons, one attached to the endoscope tip and the other to the tip of an atraumatic overtube passed over the scope. By inflating the scope tip balloon, the overtube (with the overtube balloon deflated) can be advanced over the scope. Once it is close to the scope tip, the overtube balloon is inflated to anchor the straightened position and the scope tip balloon deflated to allow further forward insertion with the scope. The process is repeated to pleat the bowel back over the scope and overtube and is ideal for unusually long and mobile colons. A single balloon system is also available, and both report high success rates when conventional colonoscopy has failed. However, using the techniques described in this chapter and a magnetic imager, we achieve over 99% complete colonoscopy without resorting to these additional instruments.

Examination of the colon

The aim of colonoscopy is to see all parts of the colon as well as possible. The images that can be obtained with modern high-definition colonoscopes are impressive, but the endoscopist may have to work hard to achieve them. The most obvious problems of colonoscopy occur during insertion, which is why so much text has been devoted to overcoming them. However, the 6–12 minutes that should be taken to examine the colon on withdrawal are the most critical. During this withdrawal phase the endoscopist must be dexterous, but also slow and obsessional in trying to minimize blind spots—suctioning puddles, irrigating any residue, trying dynamic position change, and being prepared to reinsert and reexamine each fold or loop that may have been inadequately viewed. Examination (Video 7.24) should involve just as much skill and hard work as insertion, with intense visual concentration so as to maximize the yield of even small or flat adenomas among the folds of the colon.

Examination is facilitated by good bowel preparation and the endoscopist's awareness of the myriad different appearances of colonic polyps and pathology. The addition of a cuff or cap at the scope tip can be very helpful in revealing the proximal side of folds and stabilizing the scope tip for a more controlled withdrawal (Fig 7.6). Artificial intelligence (AI) systems are already becoming mainstream to aid in polyp detection by almost instantaneous computerized analysis of the digital scope image, highlighting the potential polyp in real time by superimposing a box over it on the video monitor. Even with the benefit of new technology it is important for the endoscopist to have good withdrawal technique, as the AI can only work well if the abnormality is revealed directly to it, and without complex robotics, this still means good tip control by the endoscopist, whose aim is to reveal as much of the mucosal surface as possible.

Better views are obtained during withdrawal than on insertion, so more painstaking examination is usually performed on the way out. However, in many areas, especially around bends, a different and sometimes much better view is obtained during insertion. For this reason, when a perfect view is obtained of a small polyp or other lesion during insertion it is better to deal with it at once (snare, biopsy, or image, as appropriate) rather than have the humbling experience of not being able to find it again on the way out and thereby waste time. A convincing example to the endoscopist who doubts this difference between insertion and withdrawal is in the larger number of diverticular orifices seen while inserting around bends (so the colon wall is seen side-on) compared with the relatively few seen on formal examination on the way out.

The colon is shortened and crumpled during insertion, and during withdrawal, the most convoluted or crumpled parts (such as the transverse and sigmoid colon) can spring off the tip at such speed that it is difficult to ensure a complete view. At sharp bends or marked haustrations there may therefore be blind spots during a single withdrawal. Careful scanning and twisting movements should be used in an attempt to survey all parts of each haustral fold or bend, and some may need to be reexamined several times. At a flexure the outside of the bend may be seen on the first pass, but the colonoscope often has to be reinserted and hooked to get a selective view of the other side. Acute bends, including the hepatic and splenic flexures, the sigmoid-descending colon junction, and the capacious parts of the cecum and rectum, are potential blind spots where the endoscopist needs to take particular care to avoid "misses" (Fig 7.94).

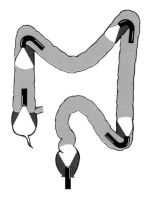

Fig 7.94 Potential blind spots for colonoscopic visualization.

Dynamic position change can help proper inspection and has been shown to improve polyp and adenoma detection and can be as relevant during withdrawal (Fig 7.95) as it is during insertion (Fig 7.14). As mentioned, a supine or right lateral position can help improve visualization of the cecum. Changing the patient's position to supine for examination of the transverse colon significantly improves colonic luminal distention and visualization. The splenic flexure and descending colon are rapidly filled with air and emptied of fluid by asking the patient to rotate toward the right lateral position. It is our policy routinely to rotate patients briefly to their back for examination of the transverse colon, to the right lateral position for inspection of the left colon (splenic flexure and descending colon), then back to the supine and left lateral positions for a better view of the sigmoid colon and rectum.

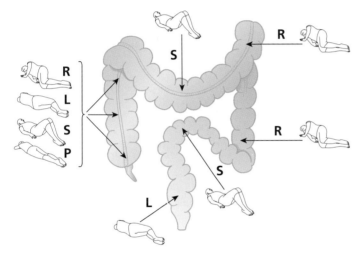

Fig 7.95 Dynamic position change during withdrawal is essential for optimal views and accuracy (L: left lateral, R: right lateral, S: supine, P: prone).

The single-handed technique comes into its own during inspection on withdrawal. The endoscopist has precise control and the corkscrewing movements made by twisting the shaft are the quickest way of scanning a bend or haustral fold so that a problem area can rapidly be reexamined several times. Using an assistant for two-person handling creates difficulties of communication and coordination that make it much more difficult to be thorough and accurate.

As well as being diligent, the endoscopist must be honest, reporting not only what is seen but also when the view has been imperfect due to technical difficulty or bad bowel preparation. Even during an ideal examination, the endoscopist probably misses at least 5–10% of the mucosal surface, and in a problematic examination may miss up to 20–30% (although large protuberant lesions are less likely to be missed). Anyone who doubts this should read both the "tandem colonoscopy" or "back to back studies," in which two skilled colonoscopists examine the same patient on the same visit, and the comparisons with CT colonography, reporting a 12–17% "miss" rate of large (1 cm) adenomas by colonoscopy.

Similarly reported "adenoma-detection rates" (ADR) vary enormously between scrupulous, careful, slower endoscopists and the "speed merchants," who should not be involved in screening and surveillance programs.

Quality control of colonoscopy is a difficult matter, but endoscopists can (and should) be assessed on their validated cecal completion rate (ideally photodocumented by appendix orifice, ileo-cecal valve and/or terminal ileum), adenoma detection rate during screening exams, and the time taken for withdrawal. Continuous quality improvement programs now form part of many societies' recommendations on credentialing and monitoring for colonoscopy. As part of this there are obvious possibilities for advanced simulation to provide objective testing of dexterity and accuracy in polyp detection in a range of standardized, simulated colons.

Quality of examination—tips and principles:
- Optimize bowel preparation to ensure good visualization
- Slow and controlled withdrawal, with adequate withdrawal time
- Insufflate adequately for views (CO_2); aspirate after segment is examined
- Dynamic position change used for optimal views
- Rotate fluid to 6 o'clock for easy suctioning and washing of residual fluid
- Examine behind flexures and folds
- Reinsert and re-examine any fold or loop that is inadequately visualized
- Retroflex in rectum
- And also consider a second re-examination of the right colon with or without retroflexion.

Localization

Uncertainty in localization is one of the endoscopist's most serious problems, especially during flexible sigmoidoscopy or limited colonoscopy, but even during supposed "total" or complete colonoscopy. This can lead to mistakes in judging where the instrument has reached and therefore which maneuvers to employ. Endoscopic errors of localization can also be catastrophic if the surgeon is given wrong information around which to plan a resection.

Distance of insertion of the instrument is inaccurate. Although sometimes used by inexperienced colonoscopists to express the position of the instrument or of lesions found ("the colonoscope was inserted to 90 cm," "a polyp was seen at 30 cm," etc.), distance of insertion does not give an accurate measurement. The elasticity of the colon makes such information meaningless; at 70 cm the instrument may be in the sigmoid colon, in the cecum, or anywhere between. On withdrawal, however, assuming a fully straightened scope, providing no adhesions are present and mesenteric fixations are normal, the colon will shorten and straighten predictably (Fig 7.96) so that measurement gives approximate localization. On withdrawal, the cecum should be at 70–80 cm, the transverse colon at 60 cm, the splenic flexure at 50 cm, the descending colon at 40 cm, and the sigmoid colon at 30 cm (Fig 7.97). The last two values depend, of course, on the sigmoid colon being straightened. It is sometimes difficult to convince enthusiasts for

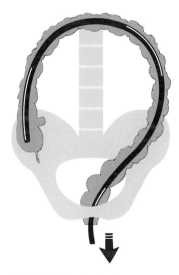

Fig 7.96 Pulling back the scope shortens the colon.

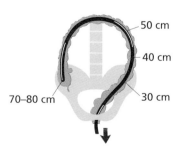

50 cm

40 cm

70–80 cm   30 cm

Fig 7.97 If the scope is in the cecum at 70–80 cm, other anatomical sites are predictable by measurement.

rigid proctosigmoidoscopy that at 25 cm their instrument may still be in the rectum, whereas the flexible colonoscope (on withdrawal) may be in the proximal sigmoid colon. Equally, it is sometimes possible for the colonoscope to be withdrawn to 55–60 cm when the tip is in the cecum.

Anatomical localization during insertion is inaccurate. In almost half the cases of a personal series the expert was wrong! In 25%, a persistent loop (spiral or "N") caused the endoscopist to judge the tip location to be at the splenic flexure when actually it was at the sigmoid-descending colon junction. In 20%, a mobile splenic flexure pulled down to 40 cm from the anus, causing the endoscopist wrongly to judge the instrument to be at the sigmoid-descending colon junction (Fig 7.62). Similar inaccuracies are demonstrated by magnetic imager series.

The internal appearances of the colon can be misleading. In the sigmoid and descending colon the haustra and the colonic outline are generally circular (Fig 7.16a), whereas the longitudinal muscle straps or teniae coli cause the characteristic triangular cross-section often seen in the transverse colon (Fig 7.16b). The descending colon, however, may look triangular or the transverse colon circular in outline. Visible evidence of extracolonic viscera normally occurs at the hepatic flexure, where there is seen to be a bluish/gray contact with the liver, but similar contact with external structures can occur at the splenic flexure or descending colon. The combination of an acute bend with sharp haustra and blue coloration is characteristic of the hepatic flexure and is a useful, but not infallible, endoscopic landmark. Pulsation of adjacent arteries is seen in the sigmoid colon (left common iliac artery), transverse colon (aorta), and sometimes in the ascending colon (right iliac).

The ileo-cecal valve is the only definite anatomical landmark in the colon, with villi often visible, but it has been stressed already that it is not always easy to find, and mistaken identification is possible unless the ileum is entered or the orifice and villi visualized.

Fluid levels can be surprisingly useful clues to localization, especially after oral lavage. Historically radiological routine was to rotate the patient into the right lateral or left lateral position to fill the dependent parts of the colon with barium (Fig 7.98). The endoscopist (with the patient in the usual left lateral position)

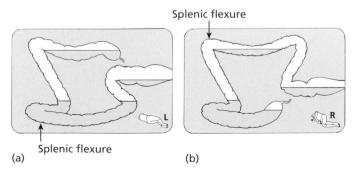

(a)   (b)

Fig 7.98 Fluid distribution in (a) the left lateral position and (b) the right lateral position.

knows that the instrument tip is in the descending colon when it enters fluid (Fig 7.60), and is in the transverse colon when it leaves the fluid for the triangular and air-filled lumen of the transverse colon. However, a long transverse colon, when it sags down, can also contain a large amount of fluid, so mobile colons are particularly difficult for localization (and everything else).

Transillumination of the abdominal wall can be helpful if other imaging modalities are not available, but in obese patients this may necessitate a completely dark room. It should be remembered that the descending colon is so far posterior that no light is usually visible and that the surface marking of the splenic and hepatic flexures is by transillumination through the rib cage posteriorly. Light in the right iliac fossa is suggestive, but not conclusive, that the instrument is in the cecum; similar appearances can be produced if the tip stretches and transilluminates the sigmoid or mid-transverse colon.

Finger indentation, palpation, or balloting can be effective, particularly in the ascending colon or cecum, where close apposition to the abdominal wall should make the impression of a palpating finger easily visible to the endoscopist, unless the patient is obese. If in doubt indent in several places and beware the possibility of transmitted forces giving misleading impressions, literally.

Location of the instrument tip or of lesions found during colonoscopy should therefore be made by the endoscopist in broad anatomical terms (e.g. "the polyp was seen on withdrawing the instrument at 30 cm in the proximal sigmoid colon"). The distance of instrument insertion may often be omitted altogether so that there is no chance of confusion in the mind of someone unfamiliar with the degree of shortening possible in the colon. Inaccurate localization can occur even when imaging is employed, and the endoscopist usually needs to rely on a combination of assessments—distance inserted, distance after withdrawal, and straightening of the shaft, endoscopic (and magnetic imager when available) appearances, and possibly visualization of palpating fingers or transillumination. Knowing the pitfalls and being careful should make localization reasonably accurate, but even experienced endoscopists can mistake the sigmoid colon for the splenic flexure, or the splenic flexure for the hepatic flexure, which can be a serious error if localizing a lesion before surgery.

Normal appearances

High-definition colonoscopes now allow visualization of the colonic mucosa in unprecedented detail and clarity. The colonic mucosa normally shows a generalized fine, ramifying vascular pattern, which can often be seen to be composed of parallel pairs of vessels comprising a venule (larger, bluer) and an arteriole (Video 7.25). The veins become particularly prominent in the rectum, notably so in the anal canal if a proctoscope is used to impede venous return and distend the hemorrhoidal plexus. The vessel pattern in the colon depends on the transparency of the normal colonic epithelium, as the vessels seen are in the submucosa. If the epithelial capillaries are dilated (as may occur after bowel preparation) the vascular pattern may be partly obscured. If hyperemia is marked (as in inflammatory bowel disease) there is no visible pattern. If the epithelial layer is thickened (as in the "atrophy" of inactive chronic inflammatory disease) the mucosa appears pale and featureless, even though biopsies may be essentially normal.

The most convincing demonstration of how poorly the endoscopist normally sees the epithelial surface is to spray dye (0.1–0.4% indigo carmine) onto the colonic mucosa. Small irregularities and lymphoid follicles stand out and there is a fine interconnecting pattern of circumferential "innominate grooves" on the surface into which the dye sinks, providing there is no excess of mucus on the surface.

Prominent vessels should not be thought of as abnormal, and are not likely to be hemangiomatous or variceal unless they are markedly tortuous or serpentine. Mucosal trauma can occur during insertion of the colonoscope, and red or bloodstained patches may sometimes be seen on withdrawal, especially in the sigmoid or where the scope tip or looped sigmoid colon has traumatized other parts of the colon. Sometimes it may be wise to irrigate or to take biopsies to ensure that these appearances are not evidence of inflammatory change.

Abnormal appearances

It is not the purpose of this book to cover more than the most obvious points of endoscopic pathology, which are fully featured in the various available atlases of endoscopy. Fortunately for the endoscopist, nearly all colonic abnormalities are either mucosal, with characteristic discoloration, or project into the lumen so that they are easy to see and excise or biopsy (Videos 7.26 and 7.27).

Polyps

The normal colonic mucosa is pale, so submucosal abnormalities are too, including lipomas or gas cysts. The *smallest polyps* (of whatever histology) are also pale and those of 1–2 mm diameter may be transparent and invisible except with dye spray. In polyps that are 3–4 mm in diameter, there may equally be little difference in appearance between a normal mucosal excrescence and a hyperplastic, adenomatous, or any other type of polyp, although small adenomas are more often redder than the background mucosa and frequently have a network of fine capillaries around elongated crypts on the surface in close-up view. The combination of high-resolution or zoom endoscopes with blue light imaging where white light is filtered toward the blue and green end of the light spectrum (narrow band imaging) picks out and enhances vascular surface structures and defines the surface appearance of polyps. The endoscopist has truly microscopic views and can diagnose small polyps optically with adenomas being slightly darker brown in color than the background normal mucosa.

Melanosis makes the smallest polyps easy to pick out if the patient has been a purgative taker, as the dusky appearance of melanosis coli (often most marked in the right colon) does not stain polyps, which stand out like pale islands, or the ileo-cecal valve.

Villous adenomas may be pale, soft, and shiny, but have a rough surface; they are commonest in the rectum.

Larger hyperplastic or sessile serrated polyps (7–15 mm in diameter and sessile) can occur in the proximal colon, when they typically appear brown and gelatinous because their surface mucus adsorbs bile. Viewed with blue light imaging they appear as pale as the surrounding normal mucosa and can have a "cloud-like" appearance often being more extensive than appreciated at first glance.

Malignant polyps may be obviously irregular in shape or contain areas of "clear mucosal demarcation or depression," may bleed easily from surface ulceration or be paler, and typically are also firmer to palpation with the biopsy forceps. Such signs of possible malignancy in a stalked polyp warn the endoscopist to electrocoagulate the base thoroughly, to obtain a histological opinion on the stalk, and to localize and tattoo the polyp site carefully for follow-up and in case subsequent surgery is indicated.

Submucosal lesions

Submucosal lesions, which are difficult to diagnose accurately as biopsy is rarely diagnostic, include lipomas (soft to palpation with the biopsy forceps and sometimes yellowish in appearance), gastrointestinal stromal tumors (GISTs), neuroendocrine tumors and leiomyomas (which are hard to palpation), secondary carcinoma, endometriosis, and a few large-vessel hemangiomas. The endoscopist may see nothing, or remarkably little compared with the radiologist, of extracolonic communications such as tracks or fistulae. Any experienced endoscopist has, through bitter experience, learned humility in visual interpretation and also takes care to provide appropriate specimens for pathological opinion when relevant. Lipomas are relatively common findings, particularly seen around the ileo-cecal valve area, rarely require removal, and can be confidently diagnosed by CT scanning if there is any diagnostic doubt at colonoscopy.

Carcinomas

Carcinomas are usually very obvious. They are larger and have a more extensive and irregular base than a polyp. Ulcer cancers are uncommon in the colon but look like malignant gastric ulcers. However, small "early cancers" do occur, typically 6–20 mm in diameter with a slightly depressed center.

Conditions that can almost exactly mimic malignancy are granulation tissue masses at an anastomosis, larger granulation tissue polyps in chronic ulcerative colitis, and (rarely) the acute stage of an ischemic process. Biopsy evidence should always be obtained, bearing in mind that the pathologist may only be able to report "dysplastic tissue," as there may not be diagnostic evidence of invasive malignancy if the specimens are too superficial. Any suspected cancer between the rectum and the cecum should be tattooed for surgical localization. Tattooing for a cecal lesion is unnecessary and tattooing in the rectum is controversial, as some surgeons are concerned that the tattoo ink could affect surgical planes.

Inflammatory bowel disease

Biopsies must always be taken in any patient with bowel frequency, loose stools, or any clinical suspicion of inflammatory disease (Videos 7.28 and 7.29). "Microscopic colitis" of any kind can look absolutely normal to the endoscopist though show clear histological abnormalities. "Collagenous colitis," a form of microscopic colitis, is a relatively common cause of unexplained diarrhea, particularly in older female patients. It is due to an extensive "plate" of collagen under the epithelial surface and also appears normal endoscopically so the diagnosis can only be made on biopsies (at least six should be taken at intervals around the colon) in any patient with diarrhea.

Mucosal abnormality can vary enormously in different forms of inflammatory bowel disease. Inflamed mucosa can show the most minute haziness of vascular pattern, slight reddening, or a tendency to friability (easy bleeding). Colonoscopic biopsies rarely yield diagnostic granulomas in Crohn's disease, whereas the appearance of multiple, small, flat or volcano-like "aphthoid" ulcers set in a normal vascular pattern is characteristic. The differential diagnosis of the various specific and nonspecific inflammatory disorders may not be easy: infective conditions, ulcerative, ischemic, irradiation, and Crohn's colitis can all look amazingly similar in the acute stage, although biopsies will usually differentiate between them.

The ulcer from a previous rectal biopsy or a solitary ulcer of the rectum can look endoscopically identical to a Crohn's ulcer, whereas tuberculous ulcers are similar but more heaped up, and amebic ulcers more friable. Ulceration can also occur in chronic ulcerative colitis and ischemic disease but against a background of inflamed mucosa. The endoscopic appearances must be taken together with the clinical context and histological opinion. In the severe or chronic stage, it is often impossible for either endoscopist or pathologist to be categoric in differential diagnosis.

Unexplained rectal bleeding, anemia, or occult blood loss

Blood loss or anemia is a common reason for undertaking colonoscopy. Although colonoscopy gives an impressive yield of radiologically missed cancers and polyps, 50–60% of patients will show no obvious abnormality, which raises the specter of whether anything has been missed.

Hemorrhoids can be seen with the colonoscope, often by retroversion in the rectum, but even better with a proctoscope used after colonoscope withdrawal. The colonoscope tip is inserted up the proctoscope (Fig 7.18) to show the patient the anorectal appearances or to take photos at "video-proctoscopy."

Hemangiomas are rare, but they can assume any appearance from massive and obvious submucosal discoloration with huge serpentine vessels to telangiectases or minute solitary nevi, which could easily be missed in folds or bends.

Angiodysplasias are uncommon and mainly occur in the cecum or ascending colon, but also in the small intestine. They have variable appearances, may be solitary or multiple (often two or three), and are always bright red, but they can be small vascular plaques, spidery telangiectases, or even a 1–2 mm dot lesion.

Stomas

If a finger can be inserted into any stoma, a standard or pediatric colonoscope will also pass without trouble, but a gastroscope can be substituted if necessary. It is quite normal for the stoma to change reactively to an unhealthy-looking cyanotic color and even for there to be a little local bleeding, but no harm ensues.

Through an ileostomy, the distal 20 cm of ileum are easily examined (ideally with a pediatric colonoscope, enteroscope, or balloon endoscope), but further insertion depends on whether adhesions have formed. As in the sigmoid colon, the secret of passage through the small intestine is to pull the instrument back repeatedly as each bend is reached, which convolutes the intestine onto the instrument and straightens out the next short segment. Thus, even though only 30–40 cm of instrument can be inserted, as much as 50–100 cm of intestine may be seen.

Colostomy patients are typically easy to examine, as the sigmoid colon will usually have been removed. The colon can be remarkably long, however, and full bowel preparation is essential. Colostomy washouts are less effective. The first few centimeters through the abdominal wall and proximal to the colostomy are sometimes awkward to negotiate and to examine, partly because of the continual escape of insufflated CO_2/air. If there is a loop colostomy the afferent and efferent (proximal and distal) sides can be examined.

Pelvic ileo-anal pouches are easy to examine with a standard instrument. Limited examination of an ileal conduit is possible, using a pediatric endoscope (colonoscope or gastroscope).

Pediatric ileocolonoscopy

There are no published data to support colonoscope choice in children. Based on expert recommendations, pediatric colonoscopy in neonates less than 6 months of age (or 2.5 kg) is best performed using an ultrathin neonatal (≤6 mm) gastroscope. For younger children 5–12 kg or less than a year, a pediatric (7.8–9 mm) or standard adult gastroscope (9–10 mm) can be used. For children over 12–15 kg, a thinner (9.8–11.8 mm) pediatric colonoscope is generally used but may be too large for some children under 4 years of age. The main advantage of a purpose-built pediatric colonoscope is more the extra flexibility or "softness" of its shaft than its small diameter. It is easy with stiffer adult colonoscopes to overstretch the mobile and elastic loops of a child's colon. The main limiting factor with pediatric endoscopes is the smaller working channel size, which limits therapeutic maneuvers. Adult colonoscopes may, therefore, be used in older children and teenagers who are approaching adult size.

In an infant, gentle rectal examination can be performed with the adult little finger and the anus will accept an endoscope of the same diameter.

Bowel preparation in children can pose challenges given the volume required and palatability. Pleasant-tasting oral solutions such as PEG-3350 preparations without electrolytes (e.g. Miralax®, RestoraLAX®) and sodium picosulfate with magnesium citrate (Pico-Salax®) as well as stimulant laxatives, such as senna and bisacodyl, are best tolerated. A saline enema will cleanse most of the colon of children under 2 years of age, but phosphate enemas are contraindicated.

Anesthesiologist-directed sedation is most often used for pediatric endoscopic procedures, whether it be deep sedation or general anesthesia, although children of any age can potentially undergo colonoscopy with endoscopist-administered moderate sedation provided that the endoscopist is specifically trained to administer procedural sedation and there is a well-trained and vigilant assistant.

Endoscopy facilities where pediatric procedures are performed should ensure availability of endoscopic equipment that is age/size/weight appropriate as well as pediatric-specific monitoring and resuscitation equipment. Furthermore, pediatric endoscopy should be performed in a child-friendly setting.

Per-operative colonoscopy

Exsanguinating bleeding is a rare indication for per-operative colonoscopy, because angiography is normally the preferred option. "On-table" cecostomy lavage preparation is used to give a reasonable view. Otherwise per-operative colonoscopy is normally only justified if attempts at colonoscopy have failed in a patient with known polyps, or where the colon proximal to a constricting neoplasm is to be inspected to exclude synchronous lesions at the time of resection.

Oral lavage or full colonoscopy bowel preparation must be used in nonobstructed patients, as most standard preoperative preparation regimens leave solid fecal residue. If the bowel has been completely obstructed, it is possible to perform on-table lavage through a temporary cecostomy tube or through a purse-string colotomy proximal to the obstructing lesion. During per-operative colonoscopy, overinsufflation of air can fill the small intestine and leave the surgeon with an unmanageable tangle of distended loops. This can be avoided if the endoscopist uses CO_2 insufflation instead of air, or if the surgeon places a clamp on the terminal ileum and the endoscopist aspirates carefully on withdrawal.

To examine the small intestine at laparotomy, in a Peutz-Jeghers patient for instance, if an enteroscope or balloon endoscope is not available, a long (preferably variable stiffness) colonoscope can be used, either per-orally or through an intestinal incision; 70 cm of instrument is required to reach either the ligament of Treitz perorally or the cecum per-anally. It helps if the surgeon either

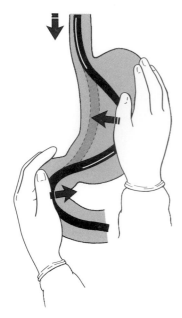

Fig 7.99 Per-operative straightening of the stomach and duodenum.

mobilizes or manually supports the fixed part of the duodenum (Fig 7.99) if the colonoscope is passed orally. The small intestine must be very gently handled on the endoscope to avoid local trauma or postoperative ileus. It is also important to insufflate as little as possible. Clamps are sequentially placed on each segment of small intestine after it has been evacuated. The surgeon inspects the transilluminated intestine from outside (with the room lights turned off) while the endoscopist inspects the inside. The surgeon marks any lesion to be resected with a stitch while the endoscopist can perform conventional snare polypectomies as appropriate. A major source of confusion tends to be the artefactual submucosal hemorrhages that occur from handling the small intestine.

Further reading

General sources

Schoenwolf GC, Bleyl SB, Brauer PR, Francis-West PH. *Larsen's Human Embryology* (6th edition). Philadelphia, PA: Elsevier, 2021.

Spada C, Hassan C, Bellini D, et al. Imaging alternatives to colonoscopy: CT colonography and colon capsule. European Society of Gastrointestinal Endoscopy (ESGE) and European Society of Gastrointestinal and Abdominal Radiology (ESGAR) Guideline—Update 2020. *Endoscopy* 2020;52(12):1127–41.

Walsh CM, Qayed E, Aihara H, et al. Core curriculum for ergonomics in endoscopy. *Gastrointest Endosc* 2021;93(6):1222–7.

Walsh CM, Umar SB, Ghassemi S, et al. Colonoscopy core curriculum. *Gastrointest Endosc* 2021;93(2):297–304.

Waye JD, Rex DK, Williams CB. *Colonoscopy: Principles and Practice* (2nd edition). Hoboken, NJ: Wiley Blackwell, 2009.

Williams CB, Waye JD, Sakai Y. *Colonoscopy—the DVD*. Tokyo: Olympus Optical (& agents), 2001. Available at: www.stmarksacademicinstitute. org.uk/resource-type/endoscopy.

Colonoscopy quality

Kaminski MF, Thomas-Gibson S, Bugajski M, et al. Performance measures for lower gastrointestinal endoscopy: a European Society of Gastrointestinal Endoscopy (ESGE) quality improvement initiative. *Endoscopy* 2017;49(4):378–97.

Lightdale JR, Walsh CM, Oliva S. Pediatric Endoscopy Quality Improvement Network quality standards and indicators for pediatric endoscopic procedures: A Joint NASPGHAN/ESPGHAN guideline. *J Pediatr Gastroenterol Nutr* 2022;74(S1):S30–S34.

Rees CJ, Thomas Gibson S, Rutter MD, et al. British Society of Gastroenterology, the Joint Advisory Group on GI Endoscopy, the Association of Coloproctology of Great Britain and Ireland. UK key performance indicators and quality assurance standards for colonoscopy. *Gut* 2016;65(12):1923–9.

Rex DK, Schoenfeld PS, Cohen J, et al. Quality indicators for colonoscopy. *Gastrointest Endosc* 2015;81(1):31–53.

Kim LS, Koch J, Yee J, et al. Comparison of patients' experiences during imaging tests of the colon. *Gastrointest Endosc* 2001;54(1):67–74.

Preparation

ASGE Standards of Practice Committee, Saltzman JR, Cash BD, et al. Bowel preparation before colonoscopy. *Gastrointest Endosc* 2015;81(4):781–94.

ASGE Standards of Practice Committee, Storm AC, Fishman DS, et al. American Society for Gastrointestinal Endoscopy guideline on informed consent for GI endoscopic procedures. *Gastrointest Endosc* 2022;95(2):207–15.

Hassan C, East J, Radaelli F, et al. Bowel preparation for colonoscopy: European Society of Gastrointestinal Endoscopy (ESGE) Guideline— Update 2019. *Endoscopy* 2019;51(8):775–94.

Veitch AM, Radaelli F, Alikhan R, et al. Endoscopy in patients on antiplatelet or anticoagulant therapy: British Society of Gastroenterology (BSG) and European Society of Gastrointestinal Endoscopy (ESGE) guideline update. *Gut* 2021;70(9):1611–28.

Sedation

ASGE Standards of Practice Committee, Early DS, Lightdale JR, et al. Guidelines for sedation and anesthesia in GI endoscopy. *Gastrointest Endosc* 2018;87(2):327–37.

Techniques

Barclay RL, Vicari JJ, Doughty AS, et al. Colonoscopic withdrawal times and adenoma detection during screening colonoscopy. *N Engl J Med* 2006;355(24):2533–41.

Bretthauer M, Lynge AB, Thiis-Evensen E, et al. Carbon dioxide insufflation in colonoscopy: Safe and effective in sedated patients. *Endoscopy* 2005;37(8):706–9.

Cadoni S, Ishaq S, Hassan C, et al. Water-assisted colonoscopy: An international modified Delphi review on definitions and practice recommendations. *Gastrointest Endosc* 2021;93(6):1411–20.

Church J, Delaney C. Randomized, controlled trial of carbon dioxide insufflation during colonoscopy. *Dis Colon Rectum* 2003;46(3):322–6.

East JE, Suzuki N, Arebi N, et al. Position changes improve visibility during colonoscope withdrawal: a randomized, blinded, crossover trial. *Gastrointest Endosc* 2007;65(2):263–9.

East JE, Bassett P, Arebi N, et al. Dynamic patient position changes during colonoscope withdrawal increase adenoma detection: A randomized, crossover trial. *Gastrointest Endosc* 2011;73(3):456–63.

Halligan S, Wooldrage K, Dadswell E, et al. Computed tomographic colonography versus barium enema for diagnosis of colorectal cancer or large polyps in symptomatic patients (SIGGAR): A multicentre randomised trial. *Lancet* 2013;381(9873):1185–93.

Ngu WS, Bevan R, Tsiamoulos ZP, et al. Improved adenoma detection with Endocuff Vision: The ADENOMA randomised controlled trial. *Gut* 2019:68(2):280–8.

Pouw RE, Bisschops R, Gecse RB, et al. Endoscopic tissue sampling— Part 2: Lower gastrointestinal tract. European Society of Gastrointestinal Endoscopy (ESGE) Guideline. *Endoscopy* 2021;53(12):1261–73.

Rex DK. Colonoscopic withdrawal technique is associated with adenoma miss rates. *Gastrointest Endosc* 2000;51(1):33–6.

Shah SG, Brooker JC, Williams CB, et al. Effect of magnetic endoscope imaging on colonoscopy performance: A randomised controlled trial. *Lancet* 2000;356(9243):1718–22.

Shah SG, Brooker JC, Williams CB, et al. The variable stiffness colonoscope: Assessment of efficacy by magnetic endoscope imaging. *Gastrointest Endosc* 2002;56(2):195–201.

Adverse events

Kothari ST, Huang RJ, Shaukat A, et al. ASGE review of adverse events in colonoscopy. *Gastrointest Endosc* 2019;90(6):863–76.

Oakland K, Chadwick G, East J, et al. Diagnosis and management of acute lower gastrointestinal bleeding: Guidelines from the British Society of Gastroenterology. *Gut* 2019;68(5):776–89.

Paspatis GA, Arvanitakis M, Dumonceau JM, et al. Diagnosis and management of iatrogenic endoscopic perforations: European Society of Gastrointestinal Endoscopy (ESGE) Position Statement—Update 2020. *Endoscopy* 2020; 2(9):792–810.

Chapter video clips (www.wiley.com/go/cottonwilliams8e)

Video 7.1 History of colonoscopy
Video 7.2 Variable shaft stiffness
Video 7.3 Water-assisted colonoscopy
Video 7.4 ScopeGuide® magnetic imager: The principles
Video 7.5 Embryology of the colon
Video 7.6 Position change
Video 7.7 Insertion and handling of the colonoscope
Video 7.8 Steering the colonoscope
Video 7.9 Magnetic imager: An easy spiral loop
Video 7.10 Sigmoid loops
Video 7.11 Magnetic imager: Short and long "N"-loops
Video 7.12 Magnetic imager: "Alpha" spiral loops
Video 7.13 Magnetic imager: "Lateral view" spiral loop
Video 7.14 Magnetic imager: Flat "S"-loop in a long sigmoid
Video 7.15 Transferring shaft loops to the umbilical
Video 7.16 Descending colon
Video 7.17 Splenic flexure
Video 7.18 Transverse colon
Video 7.19 Magnetic imager: Shortening transverse loops
Video 7.20 Magnetic imager: Deep transverse loops
Video 7.21 Magnetic imager: "Gamma" looping of the transverse colon
Video 7.22 Hepatic flexure
Video 7.23 Ileo-cecal valve
Video 7.24 Examination of the colon
Video 7.25 Normal appearances
Video 7.26 Abnormal appearances
Video 7.27 Post-surgical appearances
Video 7.28 Infective colitis
Video 7.29 Crohn's disease

CHAPTER 8
Therapeutic Colonoscopy

Colonoscopy has an increasing therapeutic role and all aspiring co-lonoscopists must have a basic grasp of therapeutic interventions. Polypectomy, in particular, is a fundamental part of therapeutic colonoscopy. This chapter covers pre-procedure aspects including consent and risks, required equipment, principles of polyp electrosurgery, and the approach to managing small polyps as well as stalked and sessile polyps. Management of very large, sessile, or possibly malignant polyps, using advanced techniques such as endoscopic mucosal resection (EMR) and endoscopic submucosal dissection (ESD) or even full-thickness excision can require special expertise but is outlined along with balloon dilatation of strictures, thermal ablation of angiodysplasias, and volvulus or pseudo-obstruction decompression.

Equipment

The equipment requirements for endoscopic polypectomy are few, and in many ways the fewer the better. It adds significantly to safety to be completely familiar with one electrosurgical unit and only a few accessories, as from this familiarity it becomes easy to recognize when polypectomy is going right and when it is not.

Snare loops
Several makes of snare loop are available. Wire thickness and loop shape affect control of polypectomy. Many endoscopists prefer to use a standard larger snare (25 mm diameter), and a "mini-snare" (9–10 mm diameter) for smaller polyps (Fig 8.1). The choice is mainly a matter of personal preference. Recently, dedicated "cold snares" have been developed. These have no electrosurgical connection, are small (9–10 mm diameter), and have a thin, semi-stiff wire, ideal for capturing small areas of mucosa. The polyp and surrounding 1–2 mm of normal tissue are mechanically "cheese-wired" by snare closure. Cold snare polypectomy using these dedicated snares, even in older co-morbid patients, is very safe, with low rates of delayed bleeding and practically no risk of perforation. Therefore, there has been a trend to use cold snares wherever possible and, in general, they are used for >90% of all polypectomies. Even larger polyps, particularly sessile serrated polyps or flat,

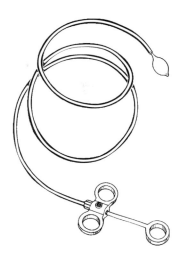

Fig 8.1 Use one commercial snare type for familiarity.

Cotton and Williams' Practical Gastrointestinal Endoscopy: The Fundamentals, Eighth Edition.
Catharine M. Walsh, Ahmir Ahmad, Brian P. Saunders, Jonathan Cohen, Peter B. Cotton, and Christopher B. Williams.
© 2024 John Wiley & Sons Ltd. Published 2024 by John Wiley & Sons Ltd.
Companion website: www.wiley.com/go/cottonwilliams8e

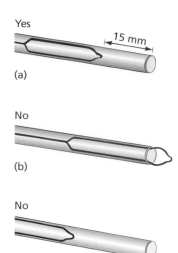

Yes

(a)

No

(b)

No

(c)

Fig 8.2 (a) Appropriate snare closure with the wire loop 15mm into the outer tube; (b) wire too loose; (c) wire too tight.

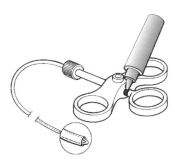

Fig 8.3 Mark the handle when the loop is fully closed.

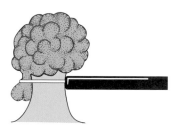

Fig 8.4 Polyp tissue can be trapped in the snare, reducing its efficiency.

benign-appearing adenomas, can be resected by cold piecemeal resection.

With any snare there are several points that should be checked *before* starting polypectomy:

1 *A smooth "feel" is essential for safety.* The snare handle and wire should open and close easily so that the endoscopist (or assistant) can estimate what is happening if the snare loop is out of view behind the polyp or its stalk.

2 *Snare wire thickness* greatly affects the speed of electrocoagulation and transection. Most standard hot snare loops are made of relatively thick wire so that there is little risk of cheese-wiring unintentionally through a stalked polyp, yet they provide a larger contact area, which favors good local coagulation rather than electrocutting. Cold snare loops are generally smaller and made of thinner braided semi-stiff wire to provide a guillotine-type cut.

3 *Squeeze pressure* is very important, especially when snaring large polyps. There should be a 15 mm closure of the wire loop into the snare outer tube before use (Fig 8.2a). This ensures that the loop will squeeze the stalk tightly even if the plastic outer sheath crumples slightly under pressure, a particular problem with large stalks. If squeeze pressure is inadequate (Fig 8.2b) the final cut may have to rely entirely on using high-power electrical cutting and may not coagulate the central stalk vessels enough, with potentially disastrous (bleeding) consequences. If the loop closes too far (Fig 8.2c), cheese-wiring can occur before electrocoagulation is applied, which can result in bleeding.

4 In addition, if the polyp is large, the view is poor, or there is any reason to expect difficulty, *mark the snare handle with a pencil or indelible pen* at the point that the snare is just closed to the tip of the outer sheath (Fig 8.3). This is arguably the single most important safety factor in polypectomy. It allows the assistant to stop snare closure before the wire withdraws too far into the tube and there is danger of a smaller stalk being cut off by cheese-wiring mechanically without adequate electrocoagulation. It also warns if the stalk is larger than apparent, or head tissue has become entrapped (Fig 8.4). Marking can, less conveniently, be performed *after* insertion by looking for the moment when the wire emerges from the snare catheter. Many snare handles have marker numbers molded-in or printed-on, but making a fresh physical mark is safer, because this proves that the point of wire closure has been exactly checked, and it is easier to see.

Other devices

• *Injection needles* are invaluable, whether for elevation of sessile polyps (saline, colloid, or commercial lifting solutions), to prevent or arrest bleeding (epinephrine), or to tattoo (sterile India ink) a polypectomy site. Long (240 cm) needle injectors will pass through any colonoscope and a 4 mm needle extending beyond the catheter sheath is more than sufficient for all injection needs.

• *Dye-spray* (*chromoscopy*) *cannulas* allow visualization or surface detail interpretation of small or flat polyps, and the margins of sessile polyps and have also become the "standard of care" for dysplasia surveillance in ulcerative colitis and for assessment of certain poly-posis syndromes. Dye can (perhaps more easily) also be syringed in without a cannula.

• *Clipping or nylon-loop placement devices* have an invaluable place, either to deal with post-polypectomy bleeding or to prevent it. The metal clips routinely available are too short-jawed to com-press a thick stalk, while a nylon loop can be difficult to place over a large head. However, either can be placed on the residual stalk when there is bleeding or increased risk of it, as in patients with a bleeding diathesis or on anticoagulants or similar medication. Ideally both a nylon loop (EndoLoop®, Olympus) and a clipping device should be available, pre-primed in case of a sudden bleed. As they are relatively fiddly to assemble in a crisis, single-use clipping devices overcome this problem. Large-opening clips (16 mm) to close perforations or occlude large stalks, as well as standard clips (11–12 mm) for routine bleeding prevention after polypectomy, should be available.

• *Argon plasma coagulation (APC) cannulas*, where used (Fig 8.5), can be either forward- or side-firing, depending on the direction of gas flow outlet. Either variety works well in most circumstances, as the essential step is to produce a localized cloud of argon gas over the area to be electrocoagulated.

• *Specialized accessories*, including "needle knives" (cutting wires of variable tip dimensions and morphology) and scissor knives (two opposing blades), are becoming more widely available and used for complex, en-bloc resections involving ESD of large, sessile, or flat lesions.

• *Specimen retrieval* may be with the snare or one of the retrieval devices such as the nylon Roth net (Fig 8.6). Smaller polyps or portions up to 5–7 mm can be aspirated through the channel into a filtered suction trap (Fig 8.7) or, more cheaply, onto a gauze placed over the suction connector at the end of the umbilical cord (Fig 8.8).

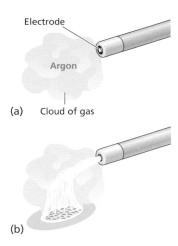

(a) Cloud of gas

(b)

Fig 8.5 (a) Argon plasma coagula-tion (APC) catheter with internal wire electrode emits argon gas cloud. (b) Activating electrosurgical unit ionizes gas, conducting current to tissue (and patient plate).

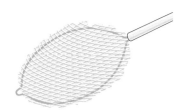

Fig 8.6 Nylon polyp retrieval net.

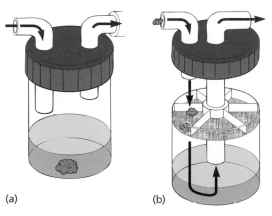

(a)   (b)

Fig 8.7 (a) An old-style mucus trap. (b) A filtered polyp suction trap.

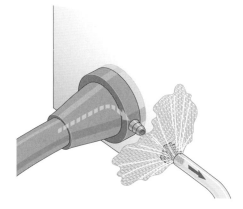

Fig 8.8 Gauze inserted over suction connector for polyp retrieval.

Image-enhanced endoscopy

Dye spray ("*chromoscopy*") enhances the view of fine detail, almost to dissecting microscope level. The principle is to spray the surface with dye (0.1–0.4% indigo carmine solution), which shows up any small polyps down to under 0.5 mm in size as pale islands on a blue background. Dye can be applied using a dye-spray catheter, usually during withdrawal of the scope. An easier method is to use 5 mL of dye in an air-filled 20–30 mL syringe inserted into the rubber biopsy valve of the scope. This allows a short segment of colon to be dyed in only a few seconds without using a catheter. Silicone-emulsion anti-bubble solution can be added to the dye to avoid small bubbles, which can look confusingly like tiny polyps.

Digital chromoendoscopy: All the major endoscope equipment manufacturers now offer electronic (virtual) chromoendoscopy at the push of a button on the endoscope head. Narrowing the interrogating light toward the blue and green end of the light spectrum tends to emphasize the mucosal surface and particularly the small surface blood vessels. Narrow band imaging (Olympus), blue light imaging (Fuji), and i-scan 3 (Pentax) are all examples of this technology. Equally, the latest endoscopes and processors enable color and texture enhancement to better define the edges of subtle lesions and to act as a "red flag" technology for flat lesions. Digital chromoendoscopy may have utility in high-risk groups where spotting even diminutive adenomas is important for risk stratification, for example hereditary nonpolyposis colorectal cancer (HNPCC) patients. Some scopes can now connect to artificial intelligence (AI) platforms to enhance polyp detection and to support polyp characterization. In the future, these advances are likely to lead to small polyps being optically diagnosed and recorded with a "resect and discard" strategy.

Principles of polyp electrosurgery

Electrosurgical or diathermy currents cause heat and coagulate local blood vessels. Coagulated tissue also becomes easier to transect with the snare wire, but this is of secondary importance. Heat is generated in tissue by the passage of electricity (electrons), the flow of which causes collisions between intracellular ions and release of heat energy in the process (Fig 8.9). The high-frequency or "radiofrequency" electric current used alternates in direction at up to a million times per second (10^6 cycles/s or 1 MHz) (Fig 8.10).

There is no "shock" or pain at such high frequencies because there is no time for muscle and nerve membrane depolarization before the current alternates again, and no muscle contraction or afferent nerve impulse. Electrosurgical current is therefore not felt by the patient and there is equally no danger to cardiac muscle. This is in contrast to low-frequency household currents, which shock because they alternate only 50–60 times per second (50 cycles/s) (Fig 8.11). At the low power used in polypectomy, even the unlikely possibility of a direct thermal burn to the skin of a patient or operator

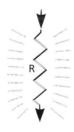

Fig 8.9 Heat is generated by electricity (electrons) passing through resistance (R)—in this case tissue.

10^6 cycles/s

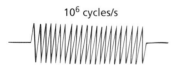

Fig 8.10 An electrosurgical current alternates 1,000,000 times per second, producing heat but no shock.

50 cycles/s

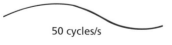

Fig 8.11 A household current alternates 50–60 times per second, producing heat and shock.

is surprising but trivial. Adhesive "patient plates" or return electrodes ensure good skin contact, and safety circuitry sounds a warning, or fails to show a green light on the diathermy unit, if proper connections have not been established. The only real danger from electrosurgical currents is their heating effect on the bowel wall at the site of electrocoagulation.

Modern cardiac pacemakers are unaffected at the relatively low power used for endoscopic electrosurgery, particularly if bursts of diathermy are kept to <3 seconds at a time. An additional safety factor is that the electrosurgical current passage between the polypectomy site in the abdomen and patient plate (usually on the thigh) is reasonably remote from the pacemaker. Implanted cardiac defibrillators, however, can be fired by electrosurgical currents, so temporary deactivation of the defibrillator by a cardiac technician using a magnet with full cardiac (ECG) monitoring of the patient is required at the time of polypectomy. If in doubt, consult the patient's cardiologist.

Coagulating and cutting currents

Cutting current has an uninterrupted (and so high-power) waveform of relatively low voltage spikes (Fig 8.12). The current flow excites the air molecules into a charged "ionic cloud," visible as high-temperature sparking that vaporizes the surface cell layer to steam. Because it is low voltage, however, cutting current is less able to traverse desiccated tissue and to heat deeply.

Coagulating current has intermittent higher voltage spikes with intervening "off periods," which last for about 80% of the time (Fig 8.13). The higher voltage allows a deeper spread of current flow across desiccating tissue, whereas the off periods reduce (except at high power settings) the tendency for gas ionization, sparking, and local tissue destruction.

Blended current combines both waveforms (Fig 8.14), some units providing the ability to select blends with relatively greater "cut" than "coag" characteristics. The differences between the various makes of electrosurgical unit imply that the output characteristics are more complex than this brief summary suggests, some appearing to provide more effective hemostasis than others. When changing from one unit to another it is therefore essential to be cautious and to start with low-power settings. If possible, try out the unit on a small lesion or the periphery of a larger one, rather than entering the "big time" unrehearsed and then regretting it.

"Auto-cut" current, produced by the circuitry of some "intelligent" electrosurgical units, will automatically adjust power output to match the resistance of the tissue being heated, the intention being to produce a predictable rate of transection. Although this may be a safety factor for some large sessile polyps in thin parts of the colon, we find that for routine polypectomies the hemostasis can be insufficient. The endoscopist also forfeits the ability to control the rate of severance and degree of local heating using the "feel" of snare closure. We therefore prefer use of coagulating current (sometimes described as "forced coagulation" in such units).

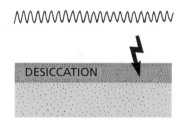

Fig 8.12 Cutting current—continuous (high-power) low-voltage pulses cannot pass desiccated tissue.

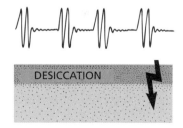

Fig 8.13 Coagulating current—intermittent high-voltage pulses can pass desiccated tissue.

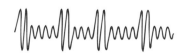

Fig 8.14 Blended current combines the characteristics of both cutting and coagulating currents.

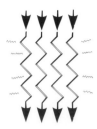

Fig 8.15 Current flows more easily through larger areas of tissue resistance and so produces little heat.

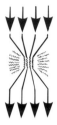

Fig 8.16 Current density results from constricting tissue and greatly increases heating.

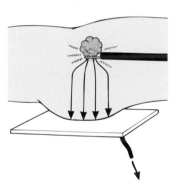

Fig 8.17 Heating occurs at the closed snare but not at the plate.

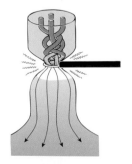

Fig 8.18 The whole plexus of stalk vessels must be electrocoagulated before transection.

Current density

Tissue heats because of its high electrical resistance, typically around 100 ohms, although resistance varies according to the particular tissue (fat conducts poorly and so heats little). Water loss (desiccation) during heating increases resistance, and the drying tissue is also mechanically harder to transect (as is heavily scarred tissue, which is relatively water-poor). If electric current is allowed to spread out and flow through a large area of tissue, the overall resistance and heating effect falls (Fig 8.15). To obtain effective electrocoagulation, the flow of current must be restricted through the smallest possible area of tissue; this is the principle of "current density" (Fig 8.16). This principle is basic to all forms of electrosurgery and explains why no noticeable heat is generated at the broad area of skin contact with the patient "return plate," whereas intense heat occurs in the closed snare loop (Fig 8.17). Even a relatively small area of contact between the buttock or thigh and patient plate is adequate. Extra moisture or electrode jelly is unnecessary at the power used for endoscopic polypectomy.

It is essential in hot snare polypectomy to heat-coagulate the core *of the polyp stalk or base*, with its plexus of arteries and veins, *before* transection. Closing the snare loop both stops the blood flow ("coaptation") and concentrates the current to flow through and heat-coagulate the core (Fig 8.18). Tightness of the loop is crucial, as the area through which the current is concentrated (current density) decreases as the square of snare closure (πr^2), thus causing a square law relationship between snare closure and increasing current density. The heat produced increases as the square of current density, so heating increases as the **cube** of snare closure (i.e. a slight increase of snare closure on a polyp stalk greatly increases the heat produced). Conversely, the fact that the closed snare loop is the narrowest part of the stalk means that the base of the stalk and the bowel wall should scarcely heat at all, which explains the rarity of bowel perforations during or after stalked polypectomy. Contact pressure between snare wire and polyp surface and thickness of snare wire (thinner wire, greater heating) are additional factors, with a square law relationship between contact area and heat produced.

Coagulation increases proportionately to increase in power setting on the unit dial (Fig 8.19) *and increases directly as time passes* (ignoring complicating features such as heat dissipation) (Fig 8.20).

Closure of the snare loop is the most important variable, because of the cubed increase of heat production as the snare closes (Fig 8.21). If the snare is too loose it will hardly heat the tissue at all; if it is too tight it will heat the tissue too fast. The soft stalk of a small polyp should, therefore, coagulate rapidly. A larger stalk, being less compressible, requires a slightly higher power setting and more time before visible tissue coagulation occurs. Visually it can be difficult to be absolutely sure of the diameter and consistency of the stalk, as the view may be poor and the wide-angle lens distortion can be confusing. The "feel" of the stalk may also be inaccurate, especially with snares having a thin and compressible

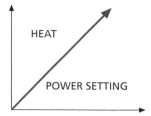

Fig 8.19 Heat produced is directly proportional to power . . .

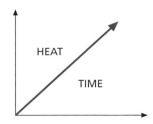

Fig 8.20 . . . and directly proportional to time . . .

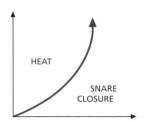

Fig 8.21 . . . but *increases* as the *cube* of snare closure.

plastic sheath, which can result in the snare handle being "closed" when the stalk is actually inadequately narrowed (Fig 8.22). It is to allow for this "crumpling" under pressure that a check for loop closure 15 mm within the sheath is so important before snaring a large polyp with a new snare type. Similarly, to allow time to react to what is happening, the recommendation is to perform polypectomy using coagulating current only, and at a low power setting (corresponding to only 15–30 W). Only occasionally should it be necessary to increase the power if no visible coagulation has occurred; extra time will usually do the job. The "auto-cut" setting of some electrosurgical units adjusts output automatically for appropriate heating during snaring.

"Slow cook" is the essential principle of hot snare polypectomy, so as to electrocoagulate an adequate length of stalk tissue before section. There should be visible whitening as the protein denatures, with swelling (or even steam) as stalk tissue boils. Remember that some tissue necrosis may extend beyond the zone of obvious electrocoagulation whitening (which is why mucosal ulceration and secondary bleeds occurred after the now-abandoned technique of "hot biopsy"). However, if all the water boils off, electrons will no longer flow through the desiccated tissue of a polyp stalk and the wire may have to be pulled through mechanically—in principle a somewhat risky thing to do, because thick-walled vessels are usually the last part to sever. Inevitably it takes a little time at the safer lower current settings to heat the tissue. If this takes more than a few seconds, the risk of heat dissipation at a distance (and damage to the bowel wall) increases and it may be more realistic to increase the power setting to speed things up. The maximum power setting used should be equivalent to no more than 30W.

Diathermy unit settings vary between manufacturers, so it is important to familiarize yourself with locally-recommended settings. The exact setting will vary according to polyp site, size, morphology, and resection technique.

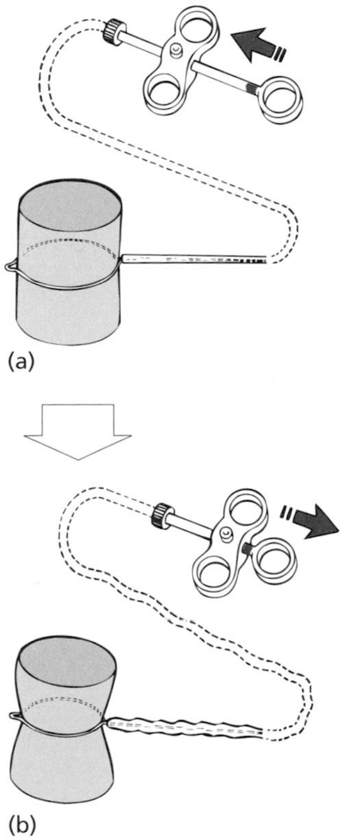

Approach to polypectomy

Informed consent and details of any medications or pacemaker must have been obtained pre-procedure (as detailed in Chapter 7). Any adult having a colonoscopy should be warned of the possibility

(a)

(b)

Fig 8.22 When snaring a thick stalk (a) the plastic sheath may crumple before closure is adequate (b).

of incidental polyp(s) being found, and the benefits of removal discussed. Patients on anti-platelet medication or anticoagulants, with an increased risk of post-polypectomy procedure bleeding, may need deferred examination after stopping the medication. For others, referred because of a known and possibly problematic polyp, the choice of endoscopist can be the critical factor, both for competence in the intended procedure and for examination of the whole colon. The risks of therapeutic colonoscopy are surprisingly low, but delayed bleeding or pain can occur after an apparently straightforward procedure or polyps found unexpectedly in a screening procedure. All patients should therefore be properly briefed before and after the event.

When deciding whether to resect a polyp, there are a number of important considerations required to ensure a safe resection without complication (Table 8.1). The first step is to ensure that there are no features of submucosal invasion, using advanced endoscopic imaging, which would rule out endoscopic resection. If the polyp has no such features, one should then assess ease of resection based on the size, morphology, site, and access. Based on this assessment, if the polyp is benign, polypectomy is within the competence level and experience of the endoscopist, and the patient is appropriately consented, polypectomy can be performed. Additionally, before polypectomy, always check equipment, including clips and diathermy, to ensure that these are available in case of an adverse event.

Table 8.1 Key considerations for polypectomy

1. Assess and obtain consent from the patient, ensuring that anticoagulants are stopped appropriately.
2. Evaluate and photodocument the polyp. Ensure that there are no malignant features.
3. Assess ease of resection (size, morphology, site, and access).
4. Decide whether to resect (weigh the pros and cons)—and perform resection only if the polyp is benign, the patient has provided consent, and polypectomy is within the competence level of the endoscopist.
5. Ensure that clips and diathermy are available in case of an adverse event.
6. Optimize the patient's position for view and access.
7. Select the method of polyp resection.
8. Ensure complete resection (treat residual polyp if required).
9. Collect the polyp specimen(s) for histology.

Prior to polypectomy, the patient should be positioned to optimally visualize the polyp and the endoscope straightened to give controlled tip access with the polyp base orientated to the 5 or 6 o'clock location. The type of resection is primarily determined by polyp size and shape, and endoscopist preference. After polypectomy, it is important to meticulously examine the resection site including the margins, with photodocumentation ideally, to ensure completeness of resection. A distal cap may help to improve visualization of the margins. Any residual polyp tissue should be removed. Finally, the polyp specimen(s) should be retrieved for histology.

Selection of polypectomy technique

The polypectomy technique should be appropriate for the size and shape of the polyp (Table 8.2). Sessile or flat polyps 1–9 mm in size should usually be removed with cold snare polypectomy, except for polyps ≤3 mm where cold biopsy forceps can be used for technically difficult cases. Polyps ≥10 mm should be assessed with advanced endoscopic imaging to ensure that there is no submucosal invasion. For noninvasive lesions 10–19 mm in size, hot snare polypectomy is used (submucosal injection can be used to reduce risk of thermal injury) or cold snare piecemeal EMR for minimally elevated lesions such as sessile serrated polyps (SSPs). For polyps ≥20 mm in size, en-bloc EMR is recommended where possible (piecemeal EMR may be required in complex cases or where en-bloc resection is unsafe). Polyps >40 mm or with a complex or unusual appearance should ideally be referred for a specialist endoscopic opinion.

Table 8.2 Resection method for noninvasive polyps by size and shape

Polyp shape	Polyp size	Resection method
Sessile/flat	≤3 mm	Cold snare; if technically difficult, cold forceps
	4–9 mm	Cold snare
	10–19 mm	Hot snare polypectomy (consider submucosal injection) or cold snare piecemeal EMR for minimally elevated lesions such as SSPs
	≥20 mm	EMR (en-bloc if feasible/safe, otherwise piecemeal)
Pedunculated	Head <20 mm and stalk width <10 mm	Hot snare polypectomy
	Head ≥20 mm or stalk width ≥10 mm	Inject with dilute adrenaline and/or prophylactic mechanical hemostasis (clips or loop) prior to or after hot snare polypectomy

Pedunculated polyps with a head <20 mm and stalk width <10 mm can be removed with hot snare polypectomy without pre-injection of the stalk. Where the polyp head is ≥20 mm or stalk width is ≥10 mm, pre-injection with dilute adrenaline and/or prophylactic mechanical hemostasis (e.g. clipping) prior to or after hot snare polypectomy is recommended.

Polypectomy: Diminutive and small polyps

Cold snare polypectomy

Tiny polyps are by far the most frequently encountered polyps during colonoscopy. They can sometimes be just as awkward to snare as larger ones, and difficult to retrieve, even using the filtered suction trap. There has, therefore, been a tendency for some endoscopists to ignore small polyps or to describe them as "hyperplastic," wrongly inferring that small polyps have no neoplastic potential. On biopsy, 70% of such small polyps prove to be adenomas, and only about 20% of those in the colon (as opposed to the rectum) are hyperplastic. Small polyps (up to 9 mm) in the colon should, therefore, be cold snared to achieve an en-bloc resection. If technically difficult, cold biopsy forceps (which open to a jaw diameter of 6 mm) can be used to avulse polyps 3 mm or less in size. Forceps should not be used for larger polyps due to the risk of incomplete resection.

Hot forceps are no longer used due to high rates of incomplete resection, unacceptable risk of adverse events, and poor tissue sampling specimens that are often unsuitable for histopathological examination due to heat effect.

Dedicated mini cold snares (9–10 mm loop size) are convenient for snaring most small polyps, opening predictably within the close-up view required. However, by coordinating carefully with the assistant when opening and closing the loop, a standard (25 mm) or larger loop can be used if a mini-snare is not available.

Snaring small polyps accurately can be technically demanding. Some skill is needed to lasso the tiny lesion at its base, and then to locate and aspirate the severed specimen for histology.

Cold snare polypectomy with no electrocoagulation is the preferred technique for small polyps due to a better safety profile, particularly a very low risk of delayed bleeding—the most common major adverse event of any polypectomy (Video 8.1). It relies on the cold snare only transecting the very superficial part of the submucosa layer, where vessels are small, and once mechanically transected only minor immediate oozing occurs, provided platelet function is normal (low-dose aspirin does not increase the risk of significant bleeding).

The following steps and points should help ensure complete resection with cold snare polypectomy (Fig 8.23):

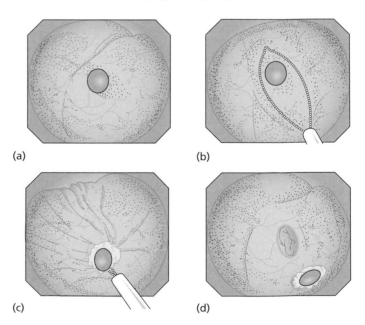

(a) (b) (c) (d)

Fig 8.23 Cold snare polypectomy whereby (a) a small polyp is identified, (b) a cold snare is placed over the polyp with a small rim of normal tissue, (c) the snare is closed, and (d) the polyp resected.

1 *Rotate the endoscope* such that the polyp is aligned with the working channel in the 5–6 o'clock position.

2 *Angle the endoscope tip downward* toward the mucosa to enable the snare to undercut the polyp.

3 *Encircle a cuff of normal tissue (1–2 mm)* surrounding the polyp with the snare, suctioning some air from the lumen so that the mucosa is not stretched.

4 *Apply gentle downward pressure* so the snare is pressed into the mucosa and the tip of the snare tube is anchored about 1–2 mm away from the polyp base to assure a small healthy tissue margin around the polyp (i.e. complete resection).

5 *Close the snare slowly and steadily*, while suctioning some air and maintaining gentle downward pressure of the snare tube on the mucosa to ensure that the snare undercuts the polyp.

6 *The polyp will generally remain in place for easy retrieval* through the working channel or can be caught by reopening and partially closing the snare to pick up the polyp followed by withdrawal of the snare tip with the polyp into the biopsy channel.

7 *Wash the resection site and observe carefully for any residual polyp tissue.* If present, residual tissue can be completely resected by repeat use of the snare or avulsion with the cold biopsy forceps.

Provided that the snare has been accurately placed around the polyp, mucosal transection by forced closure of the snare can be by either the endoscopist or, often more conveniently, the assistant. Care should be taken to slowly increase pressure on the snare during transection to feel the tissue relaxing as it transects the mucosa, avoiding pulling up a large submucosal thread. If undue force is required to cut the tissue, then the snare should be re-opened and a smaller piece of tissue taken, even if a piecemeal resection then occurs. After resection, minor oozing is expected and is generally self-limited.

Aspiration into a suction trap (Fig 8.7) is a convenient way of managing polyps up to 5–7 mm in diameter. A piece of gauze in the suction line is cheaper and just as effective for single polyps, the endoscopist being made aware that the specimen has arrived in the gauze by the silence of the blocked suction line (Fig 8.8). Larger specimens usually impact at the opening of the instrument channel unless fragmented by the snare or in the suction process.

Stalked polyps

The following steps and points should help guarantee safe and effective hot snare polypectomy of stalked polyps (Video 8.2).

1 *Check and mark the snare.* An overenthusiastic but inexperienced assistant can cheese-wire through the polyp stalk before adequate electrocoagulation by closing the snare handle too forcibly. This is particularly likely if the snare wire is thin, or the polyp stalk is small. The mark on the snare handle indicates the point at which the tip of the snare loop has closed down to the end of the outer tube. This can be done visually beforehand or when the snare is already within the colon (Fig 8.3). When a thick stalk is snared, the mark gives a useful approximate measure of its size and a warning that there may be problems (Fig 8.24).

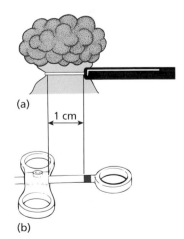

(a)

(b)

Fig 8.24 (a) Thick stalks can bleed—think of pre-injection. (b) The distance to the closure mark indicates the stalk size.

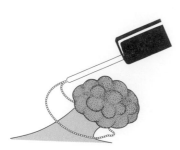

Fig 8.25 Backward snaring is sometimes useful.

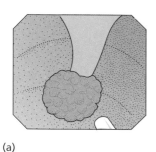

(a)

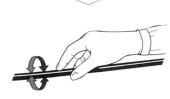

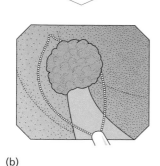

(b)

Fig 8.26 (a) Bad position for snare placement. (b) Rotate the instrument to position the polyp at 5–6 o'clock to get a better working position and view.

2 *Get to know the electrosurgical unit*. When first using an electrosurgical unit, start with the lowest dial setting and use initial bursts of 1–2 seconds at each increased setting. Discover the lowest dial setting that causes visible controlled electrocoagulation in the smallest stalk.

3 *Develop a standard routine for hot snare polypectomy* and always follow it. Check the connections, plate position, and electrosurgical unit settings before each polypectomy. Ideally the electrosurgical unit should be positioned opposite the endoscopist so that the settings can be checked easily at a glance. Make sure that the foot pedal is in a convenient position, preferably where it can be felt with the foot without having to look down to search for it at the crucial moment after the polyp is grasped. A polyp can suddenly shift if the patient moves or coughs. We recommend that the endoscope water-wash pedal (also essential to maintain visualization should bleeding occur post polypectomy) be placed by the non-dominant foot (left for right-footers) and the diathermy pedals (yellow and blue pedals) by the dominant foot, giving the endoscopist the best control possible during the crucial seconds of applying diathermy when risk is greatest (Fig 7.5).

4 *Use the closed snare outer tube to assess the base or stalk mobility* of larger polyps. Visual assessment of the stalk size can be difficult due to the distorting effect of the wide-angle endoscope lens. Comparing the stalk size to the 2 mm width of the protruded plastic snare outer tube and pushing it around to assess length and mobility can be invaluable, warning that extra power and/or longer time will be needed for transection.

5 *Open the snare loop within the instrument channel* when snaring small or average-sized polyps. This avoids the need to manipulate the snare handle when the loop emerges from the endoscope. Lassoing the polyp head efficiently takes practice. It is usually best to have the loop fully open, and then to maneuver only with the instrument controls or shaft, so that the snare loop is placed over the polyp head almost entirely by manipulation of the endoscope. It may help to open the snare in the colon beyond the polyp, and then to pull the colonoscope slowly back until the polyp head comes into the field of view and into the open loop. Alternatively, the loop can be pushed backward over a difficult polyp head (Fig 8.25) or placed to one side or the other of the polyp head and then swung over it by appropriate movements of the instrument.

6 *Optimize the view and position of the polyp* in the 5–6 o'clock position before becoming committed, especially if the polypectomy looks as though it may be awkward, which is often only apparent after trying to place the loop over the polyp head (Fig 8.26a). A change of patient position can improve the view of the stalk. Rotate the colonoscope shaft to exit the snare in the ideal 5–6 o'clock position, at the bottom right of the field of view, so that the view is not lost during polypectomy (Fig 8.26b).

7 *Snare the polyp and push the outer tube against the stalk* (the "push" technique), which ensures that closing the loop will tighten it exactly at the same point. If the sheath is not pushed against the stalk, loop closure by the assistant will tend to move or even pull the wire off the polyp (Fig 8.27) unless the endoscopist simultaneously advances the outer tube (the "pull" technique). If there is any doubt that the snare is properly over the polyp head, try shaking the snare or opening and closing the loop repeatedly to help it slip down around the stalk. Vigorous angulation of the colonoscope tip in the relevant direction may help, even if this means losing the ideal view.

8 Close the snare loop gently, to the mark or by feel, until it is properly closed. Snare closure occurs ideally near the top of the stalk at its narrowest part, leaving a short segment of normal tissue to help pathological interpretation (Fig 8.28). Initial snare closure should be gentle; the loop may be in the wrong place and if the wire has cut into polyp tissue it may be difficult to release and reposition. With longer stalks, especially if there is any suspicion of malignancy, it may be possible and desirable to snare lower down the stalk so as to increase the chance of resecting all invasive tissue.

9 If the snare loop is stuck in the wrong position, or if it becomes apparent that the polyp cannot be safely transected, releasing the snare is made easier by lifting up the loop over the polyp head and pushing forcibly inward, with the whole colonoscope if necessary (Fig 8.29). If the loop is ever completely trapped in a polyp, a second, small-diameter instrument (gastroscope or pediatric colonoscope) can be inserted alongside the first endoscope and the biopsy forceps used to coax the wire free. Remember that it is always possible (depending on type) either to dismantle the snare or to sacrifice it by cutting it outside the patient with wire cutters, withdrawing the colonoscope and leaving the loop *in situ*. Either the polyp head will fall off or another attempt can be made to transect the stalk with a new snare or endoscopic knife (or, if necessary, a different endoscopist). It is never necessary to be committed to a polypectomy just because it has been started.

10 Electrocoagulate using a low-power forced coagulating current with the snare loop kept *gently* closed to "neck" the tissue and create favorable circumstances for electrocoagulation. Apply the current continuously for 1–2 seconds at a time, watching for visible swelling or whitening. Once the stalk or base below the snare is visibly coagulating, squeeze the handle more tightly while continuing electrocoagulation, and transection will start.

11 Watch where the polyp head falls, or time may be wasted looking for it. If it is lost, look for any fluid, which indicates the dependent side of the colon where the severed polyp head is likely to have fallen. If no fluid is visible, infuse some water and watch where it flows. If the water simply refluxes back over the lens, the polyp will also be distal to the instrument tip and the endoscope needs to be withdrawn to find the specimen.

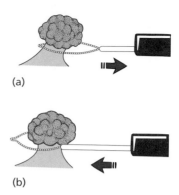

(a)

(b)

Fig 8.27 (a) To avoid the snare pulling off during closure, (b) push the loop against the stalk before closing ("push" technique) or simultaneously advance the outer tube as the loop is closed (the "pull" technique).

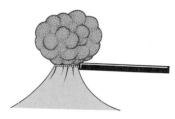

Fig 8.28 Snare at the narrowest part of the stalk.

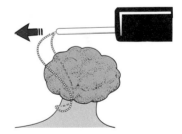

Fig 8.29 To disengage a trapped snare, push it upstream over the polyp head.

Polypectomy: Large polyps

With larger polyps, it is important first to assess for any evidence of submucosal invasion by using advanced endoscopic imaging. This ensures that endoscopic removal is safe. In such cases, techniques such as EMR, ESD, transanal microsurgery, or standard surgery may be required.

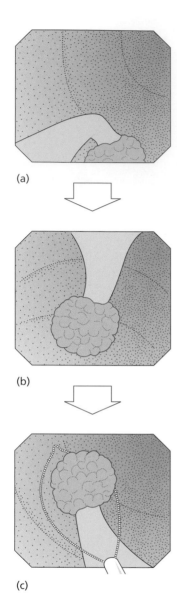

(a)

(b)

(c)

Fig 8.30 (a) Bad view of a polyp? (b) Change the patient's position to let gravity help. (c) Rotate so the stalk base is oriented at 5–6 o'clock.

Large-stalked polyps

The "large" size of a polyp is sometimes an illusion because the visual judgment of size is made relative to the diameter of the colon lumen. Proximal colon and cecal polyps thus tend to be *larger* than they look at first sight. In the narrowed lumen of diverticular disease, polyps that appear large may prove on snaring to be significantly *smaller*.

In snaring a large stalk, extra electrocoagulation is needed to minimize the increased chance of bleeding from the relatively large plexus of stalk vessels, and extra care (and time) should be taken to optimize things before starting.

1 *Check that an adequate number of appropriately sized endoclips are available in case of bleeding*, as well as hemostatic forceps, an endoloop, and an epinephrine-filled injection cannula (1:10,000 epinephrine).

2 *Palpate and move the stalk* around using the closed snare to judge its diameter, length, and mobility.

3 *Get the best view of the stalk and polyp head possible*; if views are poor (e.g. stalk collapsed), it may be necessary to change patient position (so the stalk is not collapsed) and then rotate the endoscope to orientate the base of the stalk at the 5 or 6 o'clock position (Figs 8.26 and 8.30).

4 *Place the snare optimally on the narrowest part of the stalk* to ensure maximal current density.

5 *Consider "pre-snaring" lower down the stalk* in order to extend the zone of electrocoagulation. Squeeze the snare *gently* for this preliminary stalk heating, so that transection does not occur, and the snare is easy to release and replace higher up the stalk for conventional polypectomy.

6 *Electrocoagulate the stalk* for longer than usual, until visible swelling and whitening indicate that it is safe to start transection.

7 *Consider using a higher than usual current setting*, especially if, in the process of transection, the core desiccates, and the snare will not make the final cut. Resist the urge to "pull through" the snare. The thickest arteries are the last to sever, so it is safer to raise the current setting further and let heat help to make the cut.

In snaring large-stalked polyps, complications, especially bleeding, need to be anticipated (and so often avoided). Large polyps inevitably have larger, thicker-walled, and more numerous feeding vessels. By employing a careful "slow cook" polypectomy technique, the precautionary methods described below, and the crisis-control (or prevention) accessories, the risk of serious immediate hemorrhage after polypectomy is diminished. Delayed bleeds, however, do continue to happen unpredictably, maximally in the first 24–48 hours, but for up to 12–14 days on occasion.

Pre-injecting the stalk with epinephrine before snaring may make immediate bleeding less likely (Fig 8.31a). Epinephrine

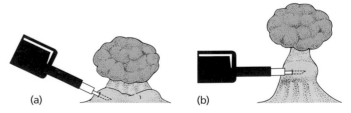

(a) (b)

Fig 8.31 (a) Inject broad-stalked polyps with epinephrine before snaring to avoid bleeding. (b) For long-stalked polyps with a risk of bleeding, inject epinephrine.

(1–10 mL 1:10,000 dilution in 0.9–1.8% normal saline) is injected at one or more sites into the base of the polyp and causes visible blanching from vessel contraction within a minute or so. The endoscopist sees blanching and swelling of the stalk, and finally mauve coloration of the ischemic head. Transection through the upper part of the stalk or above the injected area can then be made with greater confidence.

Contralateral burns are essentially a "non-problem." During snaring of a large-stalked polyp, the head will flop about, inevitably touching the bowel wall in several places. "Leak" currents flow at each point of contact, which results in inefficient heating of the stalk and the possibility of a contralateral burn (Figs 8.32 and 8.33)—often out of the field of view. The burn hazard is mainly theoretical and the possibility can be avoided by moving the snared polyp head around during coagulation, which ensures that no single point gets all the heat. Alternatively make sure that the area of contact between the head and the opposite wall is large, so that resistance is low and local heating insignificant.

During a difficult polypectomy try to keep a view of the snared stalk, especially if only part of the polyp can be seen, and ensure that adequate visible coagulation occurs *below* the snare loop before transection. If leak currents do flow up the stalk to a contact point at the head, electrocoagulation can occur primarily *above* the snare (Fig 8.33) and bleeding could result from inadequately coagulated vessels in the lower part of the stalk.

If there is any doubt about stalk electrocoagulation when the polyp head has severed and if the stalk remnant shows too little visible electrocoagulation whitening, or visible vessels at the center, it may be wise to "post-snare" lower down, squeezing the stalk gently and electrocoagulating further (without transection) before reopening and removing the snare.

Thick stalks (1 cm or more in diameter) are more difficult to coagulate, with a risk of inadequate central vascular electrocoagulation, particularly if the stalk is firm and relatively noncompressible and the plexus of vessels within it is large and thick-walled. A higher power setting may be needed to start electrocoagulation peripherally and tight snaring may also be needed to start electrocoagulation. This combination can have the unfortunate effect that, as the snare starts to transect and close down through the stalk, the heat produced increases very dramatically. This results in electrocutting of the central core, precisely the part that needs slow and controlled coagulation. Additional factors such as current leakage from "contralateral" contact points may complicate things further, as discussed later. Very large polyps with a wide stalk may be more safely removed with an ESD approach whereby the stalk is sequentially dissected with vessels isolated, exposed, and coagulated before transection.

If no visible coagulation is occurring in a large polyp stalk, check:
* *whether the circuitry and connections are correct*
* *whether the snare is properly assembled and fully closed*
* *whether the stalk has been correctly snared*, or the head trapped out of sight (Fig 8.4)

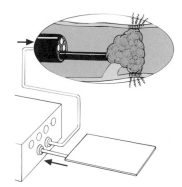

Fig 8.32 "Leak" current can result in contralateral burns.

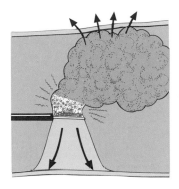

Fig 8.33 A large area of contact reduces the risk of contralateral burn, but also reduces current flow and heat coagulation in the lower stalk.

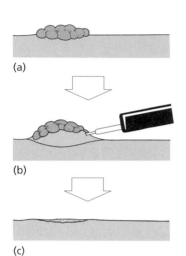

(a)

(b)

(c)

Fig 8.34 (a) A 20 mm sessile polyp . . . (b) . . . is elevated by submucosal saline injection . . . (c) . . . and snared off in one piece.

- *whether the stalk is very thick*, and if so, consider epinephrine injection to shrink the polyp head and stalk by causing local vasoconstriction (Fig 8.31) and have a nylon loop or clip ready, or consider changing to an ESD approach using a needle or scissor-type knife
- *whether the snare loop can be repositioned higher up the stalk* where it is narrower.

If there is any fear of complications or the operator is inexperienced, this may be the moment to disengage the snare and leave the procedure to someone else.

Endoscopic mucosal resection—"injection polypectomy"

Submucosal injection elevates sessile polyps for easier removal, a technique common in proctology and originally described for colonoscopic use in 1973 (Video 8.3). Injection has become a frequent routine, initially with the intention of obtaining small sessile polyps (flat adenomas) as a single histopathological specimen (Fig 8.34). "Injection polypectomy" or EMR can also be invaluable for the removal of much larger polyps, having the double advantage of creating a bloodless (when epinephrine is used) plane for transection and a "safety cushion" of engorged submucosal stroma that protects the bowel wall from heat damage. Injection can be with normal saline (0.9%) or a saline/epinephrine combination (1:200,000 epinephrine concentration), but this absorbs in 2–3 minutes, so snaring needs to be reasonably quick. To make the injected bleb last longer, a hypertonic solution can be injected (50% dextrose, a colloid such as Gelofusine®, or hyaluronic acid have all been used, with or without epinephrine). Recently, commercially available injection solution gels have been introduced that give sustained submucosal lift for more complex resections. Some experts add a few drops of methylene blue or indigo carmine when making up the solution, the blue showing up the extent of the submucosal bleb and helping to outline the edge of a sessile lesion. With a 10 mL syringe attached, an injection needle (25G) is aimed tangentially to the mucosal surface adjacent to the polyp, then the injection made by one of two approaches:
- *the "push technique"* (the preferred option) requires the assistant to start injecting *before* the needle tip jabs in and penetrates about 1–2 mm under the mucosal surface;
- *the "pull technique"* has the needle first jabbed in under the mucosal surface or through the polyp tissue, only then starting injection as the needle is slowly withdrawn.

A relatively slow, low-pressure injection gives time, if necessary, to note that a submucosal bleb is forming. The "plane of separation" in the submucosa for successful injection is surprisingly superficial and the tendency is to inject too deep, although there is no hazard involved should the needle or solution pass into the peritoneum (or the peritoneal cavity). An injection of 1–3 mL should be enough to raise the submucosa below a small polyp for immediate snaring, but 20–30 mL may be needed for larger polyps and up to 100 mL for giant hemi-circumferential lesions.

Make the first injection proximal to a large sessile polyp, so that the raised bleb of tissue does not obscure the view. Make each subsequent injection into the edge of the preceding bleb (Fig 8.35) or inject directly through the polyp surface (providing the polyp is thin enough for the needle to reach the submucosa below and there is no concern regarding possible early malignant invasion).

Failure of injection to elevate a sessile polyp ("non-lifting sign") suggests malignancy, the lesion being fixed by invasion into deeper layers. If non-lifting occurs, take no risks in attempting total removal but wait for histology. The exception to this is when a polyp is known to have been partially removed previously, with diathermy scarring to the submucosal plane, but still appears benign on endoscopic reassessment. In this situation resection may still be possible but the risks of bleeding and perforation are higher as the normal tissue planes are distorted. For any polyp thought to contain malignancy, surgery is likely to be necessary. Always remember to tattoo the site to help localization (see "Malignant polyps" section further on in this chapter).

Recently underwater polyp resection has been introduced, with water infusion and air aspiration having the effect of "floating" the polyp in the bowel lumen. While submucosal injection tends to make the polyp base wider, water infusion makes grasping the polyp easier so that lesions up to 3 cm can be successfully resected en-bloc with the underwater approach (Video 8.4).

Large sessile polyps—piecemeal resection

Even very large sessile polyps can usually be removed endoscopically, but this may require special skills and should be a matter of expert opinion and clinical judgment (Video 8.5). It was previously suggested that sessile polyps occupying more than 50% of the colon circumference, or involving two haustral folds, are too big for safe endoscopic removal, but opinion has changed as technical skills and accessories evolve. The endoscopic approach is the obvious one in a patient who is a high operative risk and is prepared to accept repeated endoscopy. If colonoscopy is technically difficult, it may be better to consider laparoscopy.

At the first endoscopic session attempt complete removal (even if piecemeal), because scarring will make subsequent attempts at submucosal injection and removal less likely to succeed. Injection is a significant help in safe debulking, but the main requirements are endoscopic dexterity, patience, and sufficient time. Piecemeal removal of a very large polyp can take an hour or so. Any basal remnants are easily and safely destroyed with APC followed by avulsion (Fig 8.5). Even after an apparently complete piecemeal EMR, careful assessment of the EMR defect is required to look for and treat bleeding vessels or residual areas of polyp. Routine thermal ablation of the defect edges with snare tip soft coagulation or APC is now recommended to reduce the risk of polyp recurrence (Fig 8.36d). Before finishing, a submucosal tattoo is left a few centimeters distal to the polypectomy site, to facilitate follow-up.

When the snare is closed over all or part of a sessile polyp, move it back and forth as a measure of safety; if the mucosa moves, but not the bowel wall, there is no danger. If the colon moves with the snare, the full thickness of the wall has been "tented" dangerously

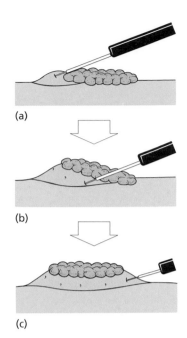

(a)

(b)

(c)

Fig 8.35 (a) First inject *proximally* to a larger sessile polyp . . . (b) . . . then around the periphery . . . (c) . . . to elevate it completely before snaring.

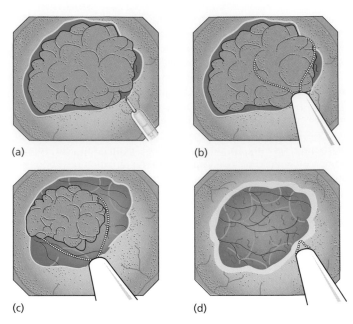

(a)   (b)

(c)   (d)

Fig 8.36 Conventional piecemeal EMR whereby (a) a larger polyp is elevated by submucosal saline injection (b–c) with subsequent piecemeal snare resection and (d) snare-tip coagulation of resection margins.

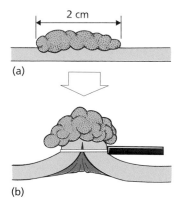

Fig 8.37 (a) Large sessile polyps can be risky to snare in one portion . . . (b) . . . because "tenting" results.

(Fig 8.37b) and the snare should be repositioned to take only a smaller part. Here the mark on the snare is also important: if the snare can be closed easily to the mark and there is a soft or spongy feel on further compression of the snare loop, the muscle layer is unlikely to have been caught and resection can proceed.

It is difficult to achieve "current density" for localized heating when snaring a large sessile (or broad-based) polyp. This is why removal of these polyps (Fig 8.37) present problems for the endoscopist and why piecemeal removal can be the safer option. For such lesions, "auto-cut" electrosurgical units may be an advance, because they provide the high power needed to start transection but reduce it rapidly to safer levels thereafter. Fortunately, many so-called "sessile" polyps up to 10–15 mm in diameter are simply "semi-pedunculated" or, if "broad-based," can be pulled up by the snare onto an adequate and compressible pseudo-stalk. If there is any doubt, submucosal injection is used to elevate the polyp tissue before snaring and sessile or flat polyps up to 20 mm in size can be resected en-bloc with larger lesions requiring a piecemeal approach (Figs 8.34 and 8.36; Videos 8.3 and 8.5).

A pediatric endoscope can be used in retroversion to pre-inject or snare the proximal part of a polyp if it proves to be difficult to see or target. Standard polypectomy snares sometimes slip off the moist and domed pre-injected area, whereas a stiffer thin monofilament snare can be effective for cutting into the polyp or the bleb beneath it. A "needle-knife" can be a useful adjunct to pre-cut around the injected and raised polyp margin, allowing the snare to grip it better and to ensure a polyp-free lateral margin. A spike-tipped snare can fix the tip of the snare into the mucosal surface at an appropriate point, making opening and control of the loop easier. The tip of a standard snare can be similarly anchored by (very brief) electrocoagulation of the tip, fixing it into mucosa.

Pain during sessile polypectomy, unless due to overinsufflation, is a warning that full-thickness heating of the bowel wall is occurring, activating peritoneal pain receptors. If pain occurs and deflation does *not* stop it (it is easy to be overenthusiastic with the air button when trying to keep a good view during a problematic polypectomy), the procedure should be abandoned until another session at least 3 weeks later, when healing should have occurred, and the area can be properly assessed.

Large polyps and endoscopic submucosal dissection

Consider flexible endoscopic removal of large sessile polyps in the rectum. Sessile polyps up to 12 cm from the anal verge are extraperitoneal (below the peritoneal reflection), so are relatively safe from perforation. They can be removed by local proctological techniques, which often produce a single large specimen for optimal histology, rather than the chaos of fragments resulting from endoscopic piecemeal snaring. *Transanal microsurgery* (TEMS) under anesthesia potentially allows anal dilation and a two-handed approach for injection, scissor-excision, or full-thickness removal if malignancy is suspected, but the technique is expensive and not widely available. The ESD technique is an attractive alternative endoscopic approach for large sessile lesions, particularly in the rectum and in skilled hands. The technique is adapted from Japanese approaches to endoscopic treatment of early gastric cancer, which can be removed en-bloc using a combination of submucosal injection and "free-hand" dissection using a variety of electrosurgical knives. The technique is slow, however, and technically demanding, so should be left to experts with appropriate experience.

As already stated, a failed initial endoscopic attempt to remove such rectal polyps forms scar tissue, which then greatly hinders any subsequent attempt at submucosal excision, so the endoscopist's decision to refer to an appropriate expert (whether for EMR, ESD, or local transanal surgery) should be made mainly on the basis of visual endoscopic assessment, complemented by cross-sectional imaging (pelvic MRI, ideally) and/or transrectal ultrasound.

Submucosal injection for EMR or ESD in the rectum should be with no higher a concentration than 1:200,000 epinephrine solution because there is risk of communication to the systemic circulation and serious cardiac dysrhythmia. Equally, give a broad-spectrum antibiotic to cover more extensive low rectal resections as there is a risk of direct translocation of bacteria into the systemic circulation with bacteremia, particularly in those with significant comorbidity or immunosuppression.

Smaller rectal polyps close to the anal canal can be snared in retroversion after local anesthetic injection (typically with 3–5 mL of 1% lignocaine solution, but without epinephrine for safety reasons). The distal 3–5 cm of the rectal ampulla is otherwise difficult to visualize properly and is also richly supplied with sensory nerves,

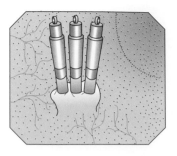

(a)

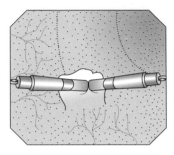

(b)

Fig 8.38 (a) Clips across top of stalk. (b) Clips placed perpendicular to stalk.

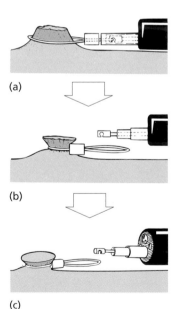

(a)

(b)

(c)

Fig 8.39 (a) A nylon self-retaining loop can be placed over a large stalk . . . (b) . . . and its self-retaining cuff tightened; (c) . . . and the loop unhooked, leaving the stalk strangulated.

a heat burn causing the same pain as it would on exterior skin. If the polyp is very small and quick to snare, "cold-snaring" may be the best approach.

Avoid the trap of snaring internal hemorrhoids (or localized varices) in the distal rectum, which can result in highly impressive bleeding.

Metal clips or nylon loops are particularly relevant to large-stalked polyps or, in patients on anticoagulants or aspirin, as a way of compressing the remaining stalk. Clipping the stalk is commonly employed and can be done quickly and efficiently, often with several clips placed sequentially across the cut stalk tip or at varying angles across the stalk to compress any larger vessels (Fig 8.38 and Video 8.6). The nylon loop (Fig 8.39) is usually deployed on the stalk remnant *after* polypectomy, because the floppy loop is difficult to maneuver over a polyp head of 20 mm or more and may get in the way of snare placement.

Polypectomy: Problem polyps

Polyps with poor access

Even an expert can have difficulty snaring some polyps. A beginner, unskilled in handling the colonoscope, can miss seeing them or get inadequate views of the polyp due to poor access, resulting in unsafe or incomplete snaring. Good polyp access allows a stable endoscope position and good views to facilitate polypectomy. To achieve this, it is important for the endoscopist to straighten the endoscope shaft to avoid paradoxical movements caused by colonoscope loops. The mucosa should be clean with any residual stool washed and fluid pools suctioned. Then orient the base of the polyp with the colonoscope working channel at the 5–6 o'clock position to optimize the angle at which the snare or forceps exits the colonoscope. In cases where access is made difficult due to a polyp being located on a fold, elevation with submucosal saline injection can enhance access and facilitate polypectomy. Changing the patient's position may also improve visibility.

Difficult sites for polypectomy

When polyps are situated within or close to diverticula, in the appendiceal orifice, or adjacent to the ileocecal valve, the risks of polypectomy, including incomplete resection and perforation, may be increased. Polypectomy should only be attempted here by an experienced endoscopist and in some cases endoscopic therapy may not be possible.

In some instances standard polypectomy techniques cannot be used as it is difficult to gain full access, such as those in the appendix orifice or covering diverticular openings. In these cases, en-bloc resection of lesions up to 3 cm with full thickness resection is now possible in specialist hands using a full thickness resection device (FTRD®). This technique also has particular utility in managing heavily scarred recurrent polyps and small early cancers in patients unfit for conventional surgery. FTRD uses a special elongated cap placed at the endoscope tip with a large, opened memory-metal clip and pre-placed snare. The tissue for resection is pulled with a grasping forceps into the cap through the jaws of the clip, which is then fired, capturing and sealing the full bowel wall thickness, and allowing the snare to excise the captured tissue without perforation.

Malignant polyps

Malignancy may be suspected if a polyp is irregular, ulcerated (0–IIc Paris classification), firm to palpation, thick-stalked, or fails to lift with submucosal injection (non-lifting sign). Close inspection of pit pattern with dye (Kudo classification type V) or absent vascular pattern with NBI (NICE type 3) should alert the endoscopist to the possibility of invasive malignancy. If doubt remains regarding the suitability of endoscopic resection, endoscopic ultrasound (EUS) can be employed, although many endoscopists take a pragmatic approach by assessing the lifting characteristics and aim to resect if lifting is adequate. If a pedunculated "polyp cancer" is possible, it is important to be certain that transection is made low down the stalk (to allow the pathologist proper assessment) and to ensure that any invasion within the stalk has been removed, without risking perforation. The pathologist should report, on the basis of multiple vertical cross sections, whether or not the polyp has been completely removed, but the endoscopist's opinion as to whether removal has been complete is also important and should be recorded. If necessary, an early repeat examination can be made, preferably within 2 weeks while there is visible healing ulceration to indicate the polypectomy site (and allow biopsy and tattooing). Because of the possibility of malignancy, each polyp is ideally retrieved and identified separately on an anatomical "colon map" in a biopsy book kept available in each endoscopy room. It is inadequate to say that a polyp was removed at "70 cm from the anus" because this might equally represent the mid-sigmoid colon or cecum.

Tattooing should mark the site of any suspicious or partially removed polyp, whether for follow-up or possible surgery. A solution of suspended sterile carbon particles (commercially available in a syringe as SPOT®) is injected intramucosally (Fig 8.40 and Video 8.7). A volume of 1 mL just distal (anal) to the polypectomy site may be sufficient for endoscopic follow-up but, if surgery or laparoscopy is a possibility, making two to three tattoos on colonic mucosa circumferentially should ensure easy visibility at surgery regardless of which way the bowel is lying. Tattoos are not generally necessary or recommended for rectal lesions, as surgical tissue planes may be disrupted by fibrosis induced by the ink. The problem of ink leakage and "blackout" of the endoscopic view can be avoided by first injecting a small saline bleb (or blebs) submucosally, and then changing syringes so that the 1–2 mL tattoo aliquot enters the bleb. The carbon particles remain in the submucosa for many years (probably for life), easily visible to the endoscopist as a blue-gray stain.

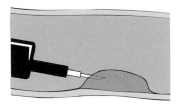

Fig 8.40 A 1 mL India ink tattoo marks a polypectomy site permanently.

Identifying adequate removal of a malignant polyp is a recurrent problem, especially if the histopathologist's report of malignancy comes as a surprise to the endoscopist. Nonspecific features of large size, induration, or irregular surface may arouse suspicion, but the macroscopic appearance of a malignant polyp can be unremarkable. The clinician or endoscopist is then faced with a dilemma but, happily, one that can usually be resolved in favor of conservatism (rather than surgery), certainly for pedunculated polyps. If the cancer is histologically "well" or "moderately well" differentiated, with a margin of 1 mm or more between the limit of invasion and the transection line, and assuming that endoscopic removal also appeared complete, surgery is *not* recommended. The likelihood of there being residual local tumor or resectable lymph node involvement under these circumstances is extremely small (ignoring the even more remote, but ever present, possibility of unresectable distant metastases), whereas the 1% mortality of surgery in older patients is immediate.

Surgery is indicated for a malignant polyp when:
- *the polyp is sessile;*
- *invasion extends histologically within 1 mm of the resection line;*
- *the carcinoma is poorly differentiated* (*anaplastic*), and therefore more likely to metastasize.

Under these circumstances the likelihood of involved lymph nodes is significant and most would favor operation, *unless* the patient is considered to be a high surgical risk. Clinical judgment is involved, balancing risks and clinical factors in the interests of long-term survival. Review of the histological slides is essential and a second opinion from a specialist histopathologist may be indicated. The opinion of the patient or the patient's family should be sought and may also swing the decision. If there is any doubt, it may be difficult not to operate in a young patient, mainly for emotional reasons and for "absolute safety." In older patients the decision is not so obvious; very few patients have been found at operation to have locally involved resectable lymph nodes or residual tumor even when the histology appears "unfavorable," but some patients found to have *no* residual cancer have died as a result of the (unnecessary) surgery. Operation does not, in any case, guarantee freedom from residual cancer; there have been reports of subsequent death from distant (micro-) metastases in spite of normal operative findings by the surgeon and histopathologist.

Recovery of polypectomy specimens

The method of polyp retrieval is based on the location and size of the resected polyp, the type of endoscope (diameter of the working channel), and the need to complete additional therapeutics and/or examination of the bowel. Smaller polyps or portions up to 5–7 mm are small enough to be suctioned through the working channel into a suction trap or gauze placed over the suction connector (Figs 8.7 and 8.8). Larger polyps may be retrieved with a snare or net (Fig 8.6) or by suctioning them into the orifice of the working channel and withdrawing them with the endoscope. The endoscope must then be reintroduced to complete the examination. To avoid needing to reinsert the colonoscope repeatedly, a larger polyp may be cut into smaller pieces to enable suction through the working channel.

Extraction of large polyps (3 cm or more) through the anal sphincters can be difficult. The polyp will often fragment if excessive traction is needed and therefore a Roth polyp-retrieval net should be used to avoid this, provided it can be coaxed over all or most of the polyp specimen. Once at the anus ask the patient to help extraction by bearing down "as if to pass wind," which reflexively relaxes the sphincters. At the same time gentle traction is applied to produce the polyp (cover the perineal area to avoid explosive surprises!).

If withdrawal fails in the left lateral position, the patient can be asked to squat on the floor or sit on a commode seat, which is more physiological and (with traction maintained on the retrieval device) rapid expulsion of the polyp invariably results. A large rigid anoscope and tissue-grasping or sponge-holding forceps can alternatively be used, pulling out the polyp and instrument together.

Multiple polyp recovery

Ninety percent of patients with adenomas have only one or two polyps, and it is uncommon to find more than five. Some multiple polyps (hyperplastic, Peutz-Jeghers, juvenile, lymphoid, lipomatous, or inflammatory) are non-neoplastic, so that it may sometimes be preferable to await results of standard biopsies or representative polypectomies before undertaking heroic numbers of polypectomies, which are probably riskier than the lesions themselves.

If a patient has six or more obvious adenomas, fortunately a rare occurrence, it is essential to examine the whole colon before snaring and to be certain that multiple smaller polyps are not present (with the possibility of a diagnosis of familial adenomatous polyposis [FAP]). Looking for tiny reflective nodules in the "light reflex" of the transparent mucosal surface can highlight polyps down to 1 mm in diameter that are invisible to direct vision, but very obvious on dye spray. Melanosis coli also shows up tiny nonpigmented polyps or lymphoid follicles very well. Take representative biopsies for certainty of diagnosis, either way.

Retrieval of multiple polyps for histology is a matter of compromise in order to avoid needing to reinsert the colonoscope repeatedly. In practice, retrieval can be facilitated by using accessories such as the Roth polyp-retrieval net, which can, with care and some skill, retrieve up to three to five moderately large polyps at a time, whereas only one or two polyps can be picked up in the polypectomy snare. Any smaller polyps are snared and then aspirated into a filtered polyp suction trap or into a piece of gauze placed in the suction line (Figs 8.7 and 8.8). A "wash-out" technique is a rarely needed compromise after the snare removal of large numbers of non-neoplastic polyps (Peutz-Jeghers syndrome, juvenile or inflammatory polyposis). On first presentation of some such patients, as many as 60–100 polyps may need removal, although their histology is of secondary interest, as individual polyps have little or no malignancy potential. The multiple snared polyps are first retrieved to the descending or sigmoid colon, the colonoscope is then passed to the splenic flexure and 500 mL of warm water is syringe-injected through the instrument channel. The proximal colon is air-insufflated until the patient feels some distension and, just before the colonoscope is withdrawn from the anus, a disposable or phosphate enema can be injected through the endoscope. This ensures evacuation and passage of most of the polyps or polyp fragments into a commode within a few minutes.

Inflammatory polyps of 1 cm or larger should be removed, as sporadic adenomas can occur in colitis patients. Most post-inflammatory polyps, sometimes called pseudo-polyps, appear as small, shiny, worm-like tags of healthy and non-neoplastic tissue after the healing of previous severe colitis of any kind. They can be ignored or, if in doubt, a few biopsies can be taken to confirm their trivial nature. Larger post-inflammatory polyps have a tendency to bleed, and there may be difficulty in distinguishing them from adenomas, as they can be composed of granulation tissue or disorganized tissue remarkably similar to that of a hamartomatous (juvenile) polyp. These larger polyps can bleed surprisingly after snaring, partly because they tend to have soft bases that "cheese-wire" through too quickly compared with the more muscular pedicle of other polyps, but also because they may be very vascular. Any broad-based or sessile polyp, and especially any raised plaque occurring after longstanding ulcerative or Crohn's colitis, must be treated with suspicion, as it may represent a so-called "DALM" (dysplasia-associated lesion or mass), the most visible part of a "field change" of high-grade dysplasia. With such dubious lesions, take mucosal biopsies around the base before snaring to discount this possibility.

Risks of polypectomy

Adverse events

Bleeding is the most frequent adverse event of polypectomy—usually "delayed" 1–14 days after polypectomy, but occasionally "immediate" after transection (Video 8.8). Bleeding (whether immediate or delayed) should complicate less than 1% of small polypectomies, although reported rates for larger (>3 cm) sessile polyps requiring piecemeal polypectomy are between 4% and 10%. Hemorrhage from large polyp stalks has become rare, as endoscopists have appreciated the need for maximum "slow-cook" stalk electrocoagulation, and the usefulness of epinephrine injection and nylon-loop or clip strangulation.

Immediate bleeding is usually a slow ooze but can be an arteriolar spurt of frightening proportions, as viewed endoscopically. Every possible attempt should be made to stop an arterial bleed immediately, as any delay can result in the view being lost or in clot formation. If blood obscures the view of the exact bleeding point, high-pressure water-jet washing helps wash the clot and surface blood away to visualize the precise point of bleeding to target endoscopic therapy. Clots are impossible to aspirate, but moving the patient to improve visualization (e.g. to the right side to visualize the distal colon) is helpful, and localization of the polypectomy site and endoscopic therapy should be possible. For stalked polyps, quickly resnare the remaining stalk and apply tamponade from the snare for a minute or two. If bleeding occurs on releasing the snare, then clips or a nylon loop are most effective. If bleeding makes visualization difficult despite position changes, then epinephrine (up to 5–10 mL of 1:10,000 solution) can be injected submucosally into or adjacent to the stalk remnant. Occasionally a bleeding vessel will be visible that is amenable to direct coagulation with hemostatic forceps using soft coagulation mode. A last resort is the use of hemostatic powder after adrenaline injection to stem the flow—but rebleeding is likely without direct occlusion or coagulation of the offending vessel(s). In the unlikely event that arterial bleeding persists in spite of all efforts, the most elegant solution is to perform selective arterial catheterization and embolization. For this reason, always apply at least one endoclip as close to the bleeding point as possible, to aid the radiologist in locating the bleeding vessel. If the patient goes for angiography a surgical team must be alerted and adequate supplies of blood ensured. Immediate bleeding during EMR or ESD is more frequent and managed slightly differently, in that clips should be avoided unless completely necessary as they may interfere with a successful and complete resection. Instead, use dedicated endoscopic hemostatic forceps and soft coagulation, which is remarkably effective at stopping bleeding, even for arterioles up to 3 mm in size. The forceps design and flat blade allow the vessel to be precisely "picked up" and just closing the forceps across the vessel will halt the bleeding prior to coagulation. When using soft coagulation, the endoscopist should be careful to tent slightly away from the bowel wall and very brief applications of coagulation (1–2 seconds) are all that is required to stop the bleeding. Excess coagulation will stop the bleeding but could increase the risk of delayed perforation.

Secondary (delayed) hemorrhage can occur for up to 12–14 days, particularly after snaring of larger polyps. Delayed bleeds may be more frequent or more persistent in patients on antiplatelet agents, which normally should be stopped 7 days beforehand if multiple or large polypectomies are predicted. Persistent or secondary hemorrhage in the left colon will be indicated by repeated calls to stool and the passage of fresh clots, whereas in the right colon the rate of bleeding is more difficult to assess because of the long delay before altered blood is expelled.

All patients who have had polypectomy should know of the possibility of delayed bleeding, partly for reassurance if minor bleeding occurs. They should have the relevant telephone numbers and be told to report to hospital for admission should blood loss be persistent or substantial. Delayed hemorrhage normally stops spontaneously but transfusion (and perhaps repeat colonoscopy) is occasionally required and the possibility of angiographic control should not be forgotten.

"Post-polypectomy syndrome," with fever, pain, and peritonism, represents "closed perforation" with full-thickness heat damage to the bowel wall. It is an occasional consequence of a difficult polypectomy, especially after piecemeal removal of a large sessile polyp in the proximal colon. Localized abdominal pain and fever

persist for 12–24 hours following polypectomy, but without free gas on CT scanning or signs of generalized peritonitis. The inflammatory reaction of the peritoneum should result in adherence by local structures (typically covered by omentum or small bowel), so it is a self-limiting event. Conservative management with bed rest and systemic antibiotics is indicated, but surgical consultation is wise if the symptoms and signs do not abate rapidly.

Frank perforation is fortunately rare. Management may often be conservative, but this depends on the area of the polyp base. A small polyp removed by snare in a well-prepared bowel is obviously lower risk, whereas signs of perforation after a larger or sessile lesion in a poorly prepared colon mandate surgery. A surgeon should always be alerted; if in doubt, it is safest to operate—laparoscopic oversewing or clipping of the affected area is the preferred option (Video 8.9). Small perforations are more commonly encountered during EMR or ESD (1–3%) and most can be managed with endoscopic clips. The "target sign" is where a small white disk of muscle (the center of the target) is seen on the underside of the resected polyp specimen and a warning of deep excision (Fig 8.41). Post EMR or ESD, all mucosal defects should be examined for deep mural injury or frank perforation and, if doubt exists, clips should be applied to protect the bowel wall.

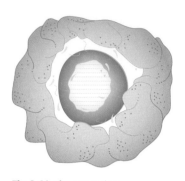

Fig 8.41 The target sign.

Safety

Any polypectomy is potentially hazardous, so adherence to all possible safety measures is essential. Assuming that the correct equipment is available, it must be carefully handled and maintained. If polypectomy is not proceeding according to plan, check the electrosurgical settings, connections, and patient plate circuitry before anything else.

The greatest single safety factor lies in a strict routine, regularly repeated for each polypectomy, because human error is much more likely than equipment failure. A military-type approach has much to commend it, with any request from the endoscopist being repeated out loud by the assistant so that each knows what the other is doing. The assistant and the endoscopist must check on each other to watch that all is in order during the procedure, having checked the equipment (including marking the snare handle at the point of closure) beforehand.

Good bowel preparation is essential to give a good view and a dry field in which to work.

Using carbon dioxide, instead of air, has not only been shown to improve procedure comfort but also prevents the possibility of explosive combinations of oxygen (from inflated air) with methane (from bacterial metabolism of protein residues) or hydrogen (from bacterial fermentation of carbohydrates).

Patient medications may be of importance. To minimize the risk of delayed hemorrhage, clopidogrel or other medications affecting platelet adhesion should ideally be withdrawn for 7 days before (to allow a new generation of "sticky" platelets to form) and for 1–2 days after the procedure. Recent data supports current recommendations that polypectomy is safe for patients on low-dose aspirin or nonsteroidal anti-inflammatory drugs (NSAIDs). Many endoscopists will proceed with polypectomy even if the patient is found unexpectedly to be on antiplatelet medication, provided the patient will have easy access to medical care and there is no social or travel contraindication. Scrupulously careful technique and due warning to the patient about the possibility of delayed bleeding are indicated.

Only a very experienced operator should undertake polypectomy in a patient remaining on anticoagulants. The patient should be warned of the possible need for immediate repeat endoscopy should delayed bleeding occur, since spontaneous cessation is less likely. Very careful precautions should be taken, including saline injection before polypectomy, and safety loops or clips perhaps placed afterwards. Often, with the approval of the relevant clinician, anticoagulants can be stopped for the 10–12 day period needed to cover the procedure and the likelihood of immediate or delayed bleeding after polypectomy. Some favor admission of the patient to hospital and switch to heparin for the immediate post-polypectomy period, but the major risk of (delayed) bleeding comes later, often after discharge from hospital.

Other therapeutic procedures

Balloon dilation

Balloon dilation of short strictures and anastomoses is easy with "through-the-scope" (TTS) balloons, especially those with an internal guidewire. TTS balloons now furl tightly enough to pass through small-diameter instruments (although a standard 3.7 mm channel gives better feel and control). The balloon is silicone-spray lubricated before insertion. The instrument shaft and tip are straightened as much as practicable to minimize insertion force and avoid kinking. To achieve this, it may be necessary to withdraw the endoscope a little and pass back to the stricture once the balloon is in position. The integral guidewire makes insertion through angulated or fixed strictured areas substantially easier, but dexterity, handling skill, and imagination are often needed to coax the balloon into position.

Balloon dilatation is best performed gradually in a stepwise manner. Start with a small-diameter balloon (10–12 mm) and increase the diameter gradually up to a maximum of 18–20 mm, although diameters of 15 mm can often provide a satisfactory result, particularly in the right colon. Short strictures are most amenable to successful dilatation but can be fibrotic or inflammatory in nature. Anastomotic strictures are generally easier to dilate and more predictable than de novo inflammatory strictures, where ulceration along one side of the stricture wall can cause an asymmetrical weakness and an increased risk of perforation on balloon expansion. Dilating balloons must be fluid-distended, using either water or dilute contrast material, because air is too compressible. A pressure gun and manometer are used because it is impossible by hand to reach and sustain the recommended distension pressures—typically around 5 bar or 80 psi (pounds per square inch)—for the

2 minutes needed to dilate effectively, especially as the balloon plastic slowly stretches a little. The gun also allows the pressure control needed for "controlled radial expansion" balloons, which give the endoscopist a reasonably precise idea of the dilation diameter achieved.

Dilation is hazardous and how far to dilate is a matter of judgment. The overall perforation rate for stricture dilation in different series ranges between 4% and 10%, so properly informed consent must be obtained beforehand, and the patient should appreciate that there is a small but significant risk of ending up in the operating theater. Very scarred, ulcerated, or angulated strictures are more likely to split under dilation (perhaps dilate to 12–15 mm initially and repeat to a larger diameter on another occasion). Postsurgical anastomotic strictures are safer and easier to dilate, especially if "straight on." Metallic stents (see "Stents" below) may have a place in managing the most obstinate and fibrous stenoses. However, the typically web-like fibrous bands that can occur at some anastomotic strictures are susceptible to "needle-knife" incision before large-diameter balloon dilation, with excellent results.

Tube placement

Deflation and tube placement is important in ileus or "pseudo-obstruction" (Ogilvie syndrome), where endoscopic deflation avoids the need for surgery. Unless a drainage tube is left, ideally inserted into the proximal colon, simple colonic deflation tends to be short-lived in effect. Different methods are available.

A purpose-designed colon drainage set is available for through-the-scope insertion, or components of an endoscopic retrograde cholangiopancreatography (ERCP) stent set can be used, cutting holes in the pusher tube before inserting it over the guidewire, leaving the tube behind and withdrawing the guidewire. Frequent irrigation of the tube is likely to be needed because of its small diameter.

A "piggy-back" method carries up a larger drainage tube alongside the scope, a loop attached to the leading end of the tube being grasped by forceps (Fig 8.42). A variation avoids using the forceps and allows better suction during the procedure (the colon may be unprepared and foul): a thin loop of cotton thread at the end of the tube is held by a loop of strong monofilament nylon passed through the suction channel; once in the proximal colon a sharp tug on the nylon loop breaks the cotton thread and the tube is free. The drainage tube is attached to a suction pump or drainage bag. The tendency of the deflation tube to be ejected by colonic movement can be prevented by stiffening it with a guidewire (Savary-Gilliard or similar steel-wire type), silicone-lubricated for insertion.

Volvulus and intussusception

The colonoscope can be used to deflate a *sigmoid volvulus*, effectively acting as a steerable flatus tube, so that the deflated loop can de-rotate passively. A deflation tube (as above) can be inserted through the instrumentation channel. However, after the tube or

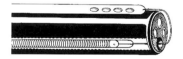

Fig 8.42 A deflation tube can be carried up alongside the colonoscope.

endoscope tip has been passed gently into or through the twisted segment, deflation alone is usually sufficient for the torsion to reverse spontaneously, so endoscopic manipulation is usually unnecessary. Only if the segment appears blue-black and gangrenous from ischemia is surgery indicated, because of the high risk of perforation.

Intussusception is easy to diagnose but usually impossible to reduce colonoscopically because not enough inward push can be transmitted around the looped colon to the ileo-cecal area (where this rare event most commonly occurs). Identifying and removing any causative factor, such as a large polyp or lipoma, should help prevent recurrence.

Angiodysplasia and hemangiomas

In treating angiodysplasia it is best to err on the side of applying too little heat. Even minor whitening and edema will progress to produce remarkable local ulceration within 24 hours. It is easy enough to repeat the examination a few weeks later to check results, but difficult to justify perforation from overaggression during the first procedure. As angiodysplasias occur mainly in the thin-walled proximal colon, great care should be taken with whichever modality is used—preferably APC because of its ease, efficacy, and relative safety. Submucosal pre-injection (avoiding the ectatic vessels) can also be helpful and reduce perforation risk prior to APC ablation. In larger angiodysplasias that have an obvious central "feeding vessel" it is preferable to create a ring of local heating points around the periphery, followed by one or more applications near the center, rather than to apply excessive heat in one area alone and risk bleeding or perforation. Occasionally Dieulafoy arteriolar lesions can be encountered, and these may be treated with APC and/or mechanical techniques (e.g. clipping, band ligation).

Larger angiodysplasias should be tackled last, and the most gravity-dependent ones treated first, because they may bleed and cause others to be missed due to pooling. The object of coagulation is to damage the superficial part of the vascular lesion (which extends also into the submucosa), coagulating the vessels nearest the surface that are most liable to trauma, but also causing regrowth of normal mucosa over the top of the remaining vessels. If several angiodysplasias are present it can be difficult to be certain which has been the source of bleeding. Surface ulceration is a rare but obvious stigma of recent bleeding; a small bright-red lesion, well perfused from below, is more suspect than a larger but superficial, spidery and pinkish one. Mucosal trauma or spots of blood are easy to mistake for angiodysplasia; if in doubt, irrigate the surface or traumatize the "lesion" to see if it bleeds. This is better than overdiagnosing and risking an adverse event unnecessarily.

Hemangiomas invariably have snake-like, very tortuous, vessels. There is great variation in colon vessel pattern, and a corresponding tendency to overdiagnose vascular abnormality. Endoscopic therapy is in any case ineffective in generalized hemangiomas, so examination is simply to exclude other lesions and document the appearance. Only the rare polypoid protuberances of "cavernous hemangiomas" (blue rubber bleb nevus syndrome) are endoscopically treatable, whether by snare excision, APC, or sclerotherapy (they can occur throughout the gastrointestinal tract, as well as in the skin and elsewhere).

Stents

Insertion of self-expanding metal stents has largely replaced endoscopic attempts at "coring out," locally-advanced obstructing tumors. The stents used are similar to esophageal stents but, partly because tumor ingrowth is slow and easily managed but stent migration is a problem, colonic stents are uncoated and their nitinol "memory metal" construction is deliberately made to be immovable (so also unremovable). Insertion of colonic stents is normally a combined endoscopic-fluoroscopic procedure. The endoscopist inserts the endoscope to the tumor, passes a guidewire above the tumor, and the stent is then passed through the endoscope over the guidewire and released under both endoscopic and fluoroscopic control. Once in place the stent expands over the next 24 hours, making dilatation unnecessary and potentially hazardous.

Further reading

General sources

ASGE Training Committee, Walsh CM, Umar SB, et al. Colonoscopy core curriculum. *Gastrointest Endosc* 2021;93(2):297–304.

Waye JD, Aisenberg J, Rubin PH. *Practical Colonoscopy*. Chichester, United Kingdom: John Wiley & Sons, 2013.

Waye JD, Rex DK, Williams CB. *Colonoscopy: Principles and Practice* (2nd edition). Hoboken, NJ: Wiley Blackwell, 2009.

Polypectomy techniques

Canard JM, Vedrenne B. Clinical application of argon plasma coagulation in gastrointestinal endoscopy: Has the time come to replace the laser? *Endoscopy* 2001;33(4):353–7.

Ellis KK, Fennerty MB. Marking and identifying colon lesions. Tattoos, clips, and radiology in imaging the colon. *Gastrointest Endosc Clin North Am* 1997;7(3):401–11.

Ferlitsch M, Moss A, Hassan C, et al. Colorectal polypectomy and endoscopic mucosal resection (EMR): European Society of Gastrointestinal Endoscopy (ESGE) Clinical Guideline. *Endoscopy* 2017;49(3):270–97.

Ferrara F, Luigiano C, Ghersi S, et al. Efficacy, safety and outcomes of "inject and cut" endoscopic mucosal resection for large sessile and flat colorectal polyps. *Digestion* 2010;82(4):213–20.

Heldwein W, Dollhopf M, Rösch T, et al. Munich Gastroenterology Group. The Munich Polypectomy Study (MUPS): Prospective analysis of complications and risk factors in 4000 colonic snare polypectomies. *Endoscopy* 2005;37(11):1116–22.

Repici A, Hassan C, Vitetta E, et al. Safety of cold polypectomy for <10 mm polyps at colonoscopy: A prospective multicenter study. *Endoscopy* 2012;44(1):27–31.

Saunders BP, Tsiamoulos ZP. Endoscopic mucosal resection and endo-scopic submucosal dissection of large colonic polyps. *Nat Rev Gastroenterol and Hepatol* 2016;13(8):486–96.

Sidhu M, Tate DJ, Desomer L, et al. The size, morphology, site, and access score predicts critical outcomes of endoscopic mucosal resection in the colon. *Endoscopy* 2018;50(7):684–92.

Tanaka S, Oka S, Chayama K, Kawashima K. Knack and practical technique of colonoscopic treatment focused on endoscopic mucosal resection using snare. *Dig Endosc* 2009;21(Suppl 1):S38–S42.

Tappero G, Gaia E, DeGiuli P, et al. Cold snare excision of small colorectal polyps. *Gastrointest Endosc* 1992;38(3):310–13.

Veitch AM, Radaelli F, Alikhan R, et al. Endoscopy in patients on anti-platelet or anticoagulant therapy: British Society of Gastroenterology (BSG) and European Society of Gastrointestinal Endoscopy (ESGE) guideline update. *Gut* 2021;70(9):1611–28.

Endoscopic aspects of polyps and cancer

Ahmad A, Moorghen M, Wilson A, et al. Implementation of optical diagnosis with a "resect and discard" strategy in clinical practice: DISCARD3 study. *Gastrointest Endosc* 2022;96(6):1021–32.

Cappell MS, Abdullah M. Management of gastrointestinal bleeding induced by gastrointestinal endoscopy. *Gastroenterol Clin North Am* 2000;29(1):125–7.

Clements RH, Jordan LM, Webb WA. Critical decisions in the management of endoscopic perforations of the colon. *Am Surg* 2000;66(1):91–3.

Haggitt RC, Glotzbach RE, Soffer EE, Wruble LD. Prognostic factors in colorectal carcinomas arising in adenomas: Implications for lesions removed by endoscopic polypectomy. *Gastroenterology* 1985;89(2):328–36.

Hewett DG, Kaltenbach T, Sano Y, et al. Validation of a simple classification system for endoscopic diagnosis of small colorectal polyps using narrow-band imaging. *Gastroenterology* 2012;143(3):599–607.

Kudo S, Tamura S, Nakajima T, et al. Diagnosis of colorectal tumorous lesions by magnifying endoscopy. *Gastrointest Endosc* 1996;44(1):8–14.

Kaltenbach T, Anderson JC, Burke CA, et al. Endoscopic removal of colorectal lesions—Recommendations by the US Multi-Society Task Force on Colorectal Cancer. *Gastroenterology* 2020;158(4):1095–129.

Participants in the Paris Workshop. The Paris endoscopic classification of superficial neoplastic lesions: Esophagus, stomach, and colon. *Gastrointest Endosc* 2003;58(6 Suppl):S3–S43.

Rex DK, Bond JH, Feld AD. Medical-legal risks of incident cancers after clearing colonoscopy. *Am J Gastroenterol* 2001;96(4):952–7.

Toyonaga T, Man-i M, Chinzei R, et al. Endoscopic treatment for early stage colorectal tumors: The comparison between EMR with small incision, simplified ESD, and ESD using the standard flush knife and the ball tipped flush knife. *Acta Chir Iugosl* 2010;57(3):41–6.

Tsiamoulos ZP, Rameshshanker R, Gupta S, et al. Augmented endoscopic resection for fibrotic or recurrent colonic polyps using an ablation and cold avulsion technique. *Endoscopy* 2016;48(Suppl 1):E248–E249.

Ueno H, Mochizuki H, Hashiguchi Y, et al. Risk factors for an adverse outcome in early invasive colorectal carcinoma. *Gastroenterology* 2004;127(2):385–94.

van Leerdam ME, Roos VH, van Hooft JE, et al. Endoscopic management of polyposis syndromes: European Society of Gastrointestinal Endoscopy (ESGE) guideline. *Endoscopy* 2019;51(9):877–95.

Chapter video clips (www.wiley.com/go/cottonwilliams8e)

Video 8.1 Cold snare polypectomy
Video 8.2 Stalked polypectomy
Video 8.3 En-bloc injection-assisted endoscopic mucosal resection (EMR)
Video 8.4 Underwater EMR
Video 8.5 Piecemeal injection-assisted EMR
Video 8.6 Clipping post-polypectomy defect
Video 8.7 Tattoo
Video 8.8 Post-polypectomy bleeding with therapy
Video 8.9 Post-polypectomy perforation with therapy

CHAPTER 9

Advanced Endoscopic Procedures

This book is, and has always been, aimed firmly at "endoscopic beginners," those in their first 1 or 2 years of training. Thus, we have concentrated carefully on the information that is needed during that time—how to perform the common upper and lower endoscopic procedures effectively and safely. However, budding endoscopists will quickly realize that the field is now very extensive, and still expanding. This chapter provides a brief introduction to some of the advanced procedures. Because of their complexity (and risk), most require extensive training and a significant ongoing commitment to quality performance.

Small bowel endoscopy

It is fortunate that the small intestine is not a common site of disease, since it has been a difficult region for endoscopic exploration. Standard upper endoscopes are only long enough to examine the duodenum (to diagnose celiac disease and rare tumors).

Diagnosis beyond the ligament of Trietz nowadays relies initially on capsule endoscopy. Patients swallow a camera "pill," which transmits images to a recording device. The biggest drawback to this technique is the fact that it may take many hours to review all the images. Artificial intelligence is starting to change this. In addition, the current capsules do not allow any therapeutic procedures.

Enteroscopes can be simply pushed into the upper jejunum, often with stiffening devices to reduce looping in the stomach. Further advance is now possible with "balloon assistance." Single or double inflatable balloons on the endoscope shaft allow the endoscopist to anchor the instrument temporarily to facilitate ongoing passage, even to the terminal ileum. Newer technology is now available that advances the scope "automatically" with a rotating spiral device.

These techniques are often required to access (and potentially treat) distant lesions identified by capsule endoscopy, as well as in the remnant stomach or the pancreaticobiliary system in patients with surgically altered anatomy. Endoscopes can also be used to examine the small intestine during abdominal surgery.

Cotton and Williams' Practical Gastrointestinal Endoscopy: The Fundamentals, Eighth Edition.
Catharine M. Walsh, Ahmir Ahmad, Brian P. Saunders, Jonathan Cohen, Peter B. Cotton, and Christopher B. Williams.
© 2024 John Wiley & Sons Ltd. Published 2024 by John Wiley & Sons Ltd.
Companion website: www.wiley.com/go/cottonwilliams8e

Enteroscopy procedures are time consuming and uncomfortable but are effective in expert hands and do allow some therapeutic maneuvers, such as hemostasis.

Endoscopic retrograde cholangiopancreatography (ERCP)

First attempted just over 50 years ago, endoscopic cannulation of the papilla of Vater was a true revolution, allowing injection of contrast to the pancreatic and biliary ductal systems to produce diagnostic radiographs before there were any abdominal scans. Its value was enhanced a few years later by the invention of sphincterotomy (for the removal of stones) and stenting (for the relief of obstructions).

The dramatic imaging developments in recent decades (ultrasound, CT and MR scanning, and endoscopic ultrasound) have almost eliminated the need for ERCP as a diagnostic procedure. Nowadays it should be used to treat problems identified by less-invasive means. It is the primary method for treating common biliary conditions (ductal stones, bile leaks, and low strictures). Its role in some other areas (e.g. pancreatitis and suspected sphincter of Oddi disorder) where it has been applied extensively is currently being evaluated by stringent research, not least because of concomitant advances in alternative approaches (surgery and interventional radiology).

ERCP differs in several ways from most commonly performed endoscopic procedures. It is performed with a side-viewing endoscope, and only in hospitals, with X-ray equipment. It is also substantially more dangerous.

Endoscopic ultrasound (EUS)

Ultrasound images of internal organs can be obtained "close up" with special endoscopes with scanning transducers in the tip. Some scan forwards, others sideways. EUS is widely used to examine mucosal and submucosal lesions and for suspected biliary and pancreatic diseases. A channel allows "fine needle aspiration" (FNA) tissue sampling and application of some treatments.

Bariatric endoscopy

Obesity is certainly a large and growing problem worldwide. Several surgical procedures are effective but are ablative, expensive, irreversible, and not without hazard. In recent years, many endoscopists and start-up companies have pioneered a variety of ingenious endoscopic approaches. These include reducing the size of the stomach with balloons or sutures and placing a sleeve in the duodenum to prevent absorption. Several methods are effective, at least for a year or two, with intriguing metabolic effects. This field is likely to expand rapidly and become a major part of endoscopic practice (until it is made redundant by a pill).

Anti-reflux procedures

Gastroesophageal reflux is also common. The usual symptom, heartburn, is usually well controlled medically, but some others are not. Surgical procedures are mainly effective, perhaps leaving little room for a less invasive per-oral endoscopic approach, but dozens have been proposed and most abandoned. These include mimicking surgical fundoplication with sutures placed in a retrograde fashion (with rather complex and expensive tools), causing narrowing at the cardia with ablation of the mucosa above or below it, and bulking it up by injecting materials. None of these methods are yet mainstream.

Third space procedures and NOTES

Having largely conquered the mucosa, brave endoscopists have been probing deeper, opening up the "third space" below the mucosa. The range of targets and possible treatments is substantial, but two have been adopted quickly.

Endoscopic submucosal dissection (ESD) allows removal of mucosal tumors in one piece, from below. Peroral endoscopic myotomy (POEM) is proving to be an effective and popular treatment for achalasia, and has spawned the development of similar approaches to other conditions such as gastroparesis.

Natural orifice transluminal endoscopic surgery (NOTES) was the exciting new frontier proposed by the Apollo group over 20 years ago. Perforate the stomach with your endoscope and you have a whole new world to work in. Advocates competed to be the first to report removing the gall bladder, appendix, and other organs through the mouth (or vagina). For many reasons, not least the effectiveness and acceptance of laparoscopic approaches, NOTES has not yet entered mainstream practice. It has, however, been helpful in that, like going to the Moon, the spin-off gizmos are often more important than the original target. The pioneers have collaborated with biomedical companies to develop many new tools that can be used through regular endoscopes, like suturing devices.

Epilogue: The Future? Comments from the Senior Authors

Old folks like to look back, as one of us did in his memoirs: "The tunnel at the end of the light; my endoscopy journey in six decades." It is more challenging to look forwards, but it is always fun to try.

The start of our careers coincided with the birth of modern endoscopy, and it has been a privilege to see and to nurture its progressive march into the heart of gastroenterological practice. As we fade into the sunset it is tempting to assume that the best is over. That is doubtless wrong. It is impossible to anticipate the paradigm shifts that could occur with undreamed of advances in technology, but less difficult to make some predictions by extrapolating from current trends. Here are a few ideas.

Intelligent endoscopes

Modern lives are much enhanced by computer chips. Our cars know where they are, how far they have been, how to get places, how much further they can go before refueling and servicing, even the pressure in the tires or when dangerously close to other objects. Driverless cars are now cruising some open roads.

We look forward to scopes being able to steer themselves or to stay automatically in the center of the lumen, know where they are and have been, to recognize what they see and report it, and to give advice when needed—quite apart from keeping track of faults and repairs and key quality metrics. Maybe they will be able to decide whether a particular endoscopist is competent, and to design any necessary remediation programs. And, while the engineers are busy realizing our dream endoscopes, they may wish to focus also on improving the ergonomics of endoscopy.

Colonoscopy—boon or bubble?

Most gastroenterologists nowadays are consumed by performing colonoscopy, largely for screening purposes. While this is clearly beneficial (as well as remunerative), it has distorted practice and compromises the consultative role for which they were trained. Currently, doctors usually do the procedures and leave much of the talking to patients to "mid-level providers" (i.e. nurse practitioners and physician assistants). In our view, the reverse would be preferable, and will likely occur for several reasons.

Although colonoscopy will doubtless become technically easier, no one can claim that it is either cheap or noninvasive, as screening methodology is supposed to be. Ideally colonoscopy should become a second-tier, mainly therapeutic, procedure for patients selected by other simpler methods. These could perhaps include capsule colonoscopy or advanced CT colonography, but, ideally, screening will be by genetic testing or cell sampling using genetic, proteomic, or other biomarkers. Eventually, we can expect pharmacological or immunological methods for preventing and/or treating polyps.

In the interim, colonoscopy is already widely practiced (independently) by trained nurses in the United Kingdom. This will happen eventually in the United States and elsewhere as demand increases but procedure reimbursement continues to fall. Of course, highly trained colonoscopists will still be needed for complex cases.

Cotton and Williams' Practical Gastrointestinal Endoscopy: The Fundamentals, Eighth Edition.
Catharine M. Walsh, Ahmir Ahmad, Brian P. Saunders, Jonathan Cohen, Peter B. Cotton, and Christopher B. Williams.
© 2024 John Wiley & Sons Ltd. Published 2024 by John Wiley & Sons Ltd.
Companion website: www.wiley.com/go/cottonwilliams8e

Advanced therapeutics, cooperation, and multidisciplinary working

Endoscopists took over a huge part of digestive "turf" from surgeons in the 1970s and 80s when the main therapeutic procedures were developed and disseminated. Techniques have been refined since that time, but new frontiers are still being explored. Endoscopic mucosal resection (EMR) has become mainstream, and pioneers are going deeper. Working in the submucosa allows removal of neoplastic lesions and also peroral endoscopic myotomy (POEM) for achalasia. The past decade has seen attempts at exploration of an entirely new frontier for endoscopy, the abdominal cavity. Many natural orifice transluminal endoscopic surgery (NOTES) procedures have been performed in animals, and some in humans. It is to the credit of endoscopic and surgical leaders that these extraordinary developments are being explored ethically and in collaboration. The special individual talents of advanced endoscopists and laparoscopic surgeons are needed.

It is a truism that obesity is a major, and growing, problem worldwide. Bariatric surgery procedures are becoming popular, at least in Western countries. Attempts to mimic surgical approaches through the mouth are far advanced, and it is safe to say that this will be a fertile field for interventional endoscopists in the future.

The traditional separation between surgery and medicine, most evident in prestigious teaching institutions and privileged countries, was understandable in the Middle Ages but is now outdated and unhelpful. Most gastroenterologists nowadays have far more in common with their surgical colleagues than most of the other "medical" specialists, and there is an increasing trend to work (and teach) in multidisciplinary groups or centers.

Quality and teaching

The recent focus on quality in endoscopy will grow progressively, propelled by patient empowerment, the drive for efficiency, and payment by outcomes rather than procedures. Is it too much to expect a day when endoscopy is performed only by those properly trained to do it, with outcome data fully available to the public? One of us has argued repeatedly in the United States (and without apparent impact) for some form of certification of endoscopists, at least for advanced procedures such as endoscopic retrograde cholangiopancreatography (ERCP). In this respect the "driving test" established for screening colonoscopists in the United Kingdom is a good precedent. "Train the trainers" courses are in vogue around the world, which helps to ensure that good habits are ingrained from the start, replacing or supplementing the traditional approach of slavish apprenticeship to a (supposed) master.

Our hopes for fully realistic and effective computer simulation have so far proved unachievable. This has principally been because of the requirements for stupendously fast processing to reproduce the interactions between the flexible scope and its accessories within the changing dynamics of the gastrointestinal tract, all necessarily at modest cost because of limited teaching budgets. Fortunately, multi-user video-gaming initiatives are driving phenomenal advances in processing speed and high-quality computer graphics, so we remain optimistic.

One of the consequences of aging is the expectation of requiring more personal medical interventions. We trust that anyone offering us an endoscopy in the future will be on top of their game (and hope that this little book may have helped in the process).

**Peter Cotton and Christopher Williams,
October 2023**

Index

NOTE: Page numbers followed by *f* indicate figures, *t* indicate tables, and *b* indicate boxes.

Cotton and Williams' Practical Gastrointestinal Endoscopy: The Fundamentals, Eighth Edition.
Catharine M. Walsh, Ahmir Ahmad, Brian P. Saunders, Jonathan Cohen, Peter B. Cotton, and Christopher B. Williams.
© 2024 John Wiley & Sons Ltd. Published 2024 by John Wiley & Sons Ltd.
Companion website: www.wiley.com/go/cottonwilliams8e